Insomnia

How to Overcome Insomnia Sleep Well Tonight

(Simple Methods and Strategies to End Sleeping Disorder)

Forrest Omara

Published By **Tyson Maxwell**

Forrest Omara

Insomnia: How to Overcome Insomnia Sleep Well Tonight (Simple Methods and Strategies to End Sleeping Disorder)

ISBN 978-1-77485-554-6

No part of this guidebook shall be reproduced in any form without permission in writing from the publisher except in the case of brief quotations embodied in critical articles or reviews.

Legal & Disclaimer

The information contained in this ebook is not designed to replace or take the place of any form of medicine or professional medical advice. The information in this ebook has been provided for educational & entertainment purposes only.

The information contained in this book has been compiled from sources deemed reliable, and it is accurate to the best of the Author's knowledge; however, the Author cannot guarantee its accuracy and validity and cannot be held liable for any errors or omissions. Changes are periodically made to this book. You must consult your doctor or get professional medical advice before using any of the suggested remedies, techniques, or information in this book.

Upon using the information contained in this book, you agree to hold harmless the Author from and against any damages, costs, and expenses, including any legal fees potentially resulting from the application of any of the information provided by this guide. This disclaimer applies to any damages or injury caused by the use and application, whether directly or

Table of contents

Chapter 1: Science Behind Insomnia

Have you ever experienced
Do you suffer from sleep problems? Do you have the difficulty of sleeping and then falling asleep during the night? What is the reason? Most of the time, sleep issues are caused by many different causes, including sleeping too little and cravings, psychological trauma and much more. Whatever the reason many people battle the enemy known as insomnia. It hinders you from getting enough sleep, drains your energy , and reduces your performance the following day. In addition, it can cause a negative consequences for your own mental and physical health.

What is sleeplessness?
Sleep issues are essentially the challenge of getting to sleep and then staying asleep. It is a description of the kinds of sleeplessness that a person experiences throughout their sleep cycle.
People with sleep disorders may be afflicted by a lack of power and fatigue throughout the course throughout the day, struggling with

difficulties in focusing on work, having severe mood disorders, and suffering from an unsatisfactory performance at work. It is possible for insomniacs to experience any of these symptoms when they are awake all night. A body requires rest in order to rejuvenate both the mind and the body. Insufficient sleep in either is sure to cause depression and fatigue. If they're exhausted to the point of exhaustion however, they fail to fall asleep or remain asleep for a variety of reasons.

The two types of INSOMNIA
1. Problems with sleep and insomnia
The first kind is the type of insomnia which is when you have only for a few sleepless nights. For many, insomnia sufferers might not believe they are suffering from the condition but it is true that they could be suffering from acute Insomnia.
What exactly is Acute Sleepiness?
The type of insomnia mentioned above isn't able to last for a long duration.
For instance, extreme insomnia can occur when those who are suffering from insomnia dealt with the rage of their boss, got poor marks on

an exam, or were disqualified by their crush or because they're experiencing a 'Poor Day'. These situations can cause the person to experience an entire evening where the person is unable to achieve any sort of sleep. A lot of people have had this type of sleep problem and also it tends to get better by itself.

2. Sleep disorders that are chronic

The 2nd type of sleep issues is known as persistent Sleeplessness. It's a type of sleep disorder that is experienced at least three evenings per week, and can last for at least three months. It usually happens when you're experiencing an extreme change in your life, either mentally or physically. It could be the result of moving to a new location or losing a loved one, moving to an office that is new, struggling with college difficulties or struggling to adjust to the harsher climate. It is possible that the reason chronic insomnia sufferers are struggling sleeping is because they are utilizing a poor rest routine that is not a proper schedule of rest.

It's a common occurrence in the modern world but modern life has disrupted the resting cycle by allowing only a few hours of sleep. In addition most people are sleeping at irregular times. They do not follow the custom of sleeping in early and waking up early the next day.

It is for this reason that insomnia is a widespread issue in our society today. What they don't understand is that their body is not capable of functioning with only the smallest amount of sleep at night, and they will be able to fill in the gaps with naps later in the daytime. At some point, your body and mind will begin to collapse and you'll likely experience total exhaustion, until you can get enough sleep. The most effective solution is to create a well-taken into consideration a timetable for relax and follow a regular and healthy sleep habits. In the event that you are not, you will need seek the help of a doctor for treatment. Most likely, it is connected to another mental or medical issue, which means that the reason your frequent sleep issues could be due to stress. What appears to be an everyday situation can seem stressful when you experience an incessant sleepiness. A shaky mind and body can be irritated at any kind of stimuli in the immediate setting.

The causes of Sleep problems.

Anyhow, regardless of the type of sleep disorders The causes are identical. The reason for this is the level of emotions the person has for a specific amount of time. The underlying medical condition can cause insomnia too. Fortunately, insomnia is possible to treat in many cases.

The medical conditions could be severe or mild and can cause sleep disorders that occur at various times throughout one's life. The symptoms include nasal allergies and sinus allergic reactions. They can also cause lower back and neck pain, constant chronic discomfort, stomach issues asthma, arthritis, and a variety of other neurological issues.

The strain and anxiety that is placed on the body of the individual will definitely cause the mind to stay awake for longer periods of time. People who contract a cold may find themselves in a state of alertness throughout the night, or wake up often. Both of these factors can lead to an extreme lack of sleep as well as rest. They may try to relax while enjoying the coolest of days, however sleepiness will definitely take over.

Physical discomfort may also trigger insomnia because the body can't get into a comfortable posture to rest. Have you had a sleepless night because you were not able to sit in the right position? If you feel any discomfort throughout your body, that is common. The best way to fall asleep and get to sleep quickly is to place your body and mind in a relaxed place in your bed. This will also aid in healing and give you a better sleep. Otherwise you'll find yourself struggling to fall asleep and take unnecessary medication if you aren't able to find your most comfortable sleeping position.

With each of these reasons to consider, we can now continue with the treatment. However, it is equally important to study all factors that cause insomnia. Did you know that there are other causes of insomnia? There is a greater likelihood of experiencing an episode of insomnia in your life, if you discover that some of these risk factors could be applicable to you. If not, be aware of your overall health and sleep routines to be sure you're sleeping well throughout the remainder all of life.

The THREAT FACTORS that cause sleep

Disorders

The main risk factors for insomnia are being woman, pregnant or experiencing menopausal symptoms, those over 40 and suffering from stress and depression, working jobs that require nighttime hours or travel for long distances when there is a shift in time or family background of sleep disorders. These factors can all could lead to a state of sleepiness.

They could choose to go on more time off in the event that they travel to various time zones. However, they didn't. It is possible to choose to work during the day, however they chose to go through the rigors working in the evening and to change to a totally different lifestyle.

It can be difficult to cope with the danger causes that cause insomnia. However, ultimately it's all about your decisions. These will eat your heart and keep you awake in the night until all depression or stress disappears. Whatever the case having the right attitude can help you overcome the emotional triggers that cause insomnia.

Since sleep disorders have a variety of factors and causes, as well as risk factors, there are a variety of options to ensure that you don't suffer many more sleepless and restless nights. Most of the time it's easy to figure out the cause however the real challenge is to figure out how to get over it, and also get an enjoyable night's sleep. The world can be tough and sometimes, it can afflict a person to the point where they're not sure whether he'll be able to get up.

The very first step to conquering insomnia is to not be afraid. Don't be afraid by any outcome or outcomes that may be expected or may not happen. Stress can cause an increase in tension but it doesn't give you. It will only increase the insomnia. Prevention is always better than treatment. Always remember to remain calm and adhere to the wellness tips to avoid restlessness.

The definition of insomnia is the problem of falling asleep and remaining at night. The first is the type of insomnia which is when you have only for a few nights of sleeplessness. The second form of insomnia is called Chronic Insomnia. The most risky factors for insomnia are being woman, pregnant or during the time of menopausal changes, those over 40 and suffering from stress or depression, working jobs that require nighttime hours or travel for long distances when there is a change in time or a family experience of insomnia. As insomnia is a condition that has many reasons and risk factors, there are a variety of ways you can take to avoid having many sleepless nights and sleepless nights.

Chapter 2: The brain of an Insomniac

Scientists from all over the world
The world is putting their minds in sync to understand the way the mind of insomnia sufferers functions. They continue to study directions of features of brainwaves in general and also how thoughts are communicated throughout the day and the evening.

How exactly the mind functions
Through the course of every hour of the day It is the mind's capacity to adapt itself to any kind of new situation. When you're trying to find food, get a drink or leave your vehicle or going through an entrance, or just get some rest, the mind will constantly seek new ways to expand and get through. It'll continue with the process of getting enough energy throughout the day and having enough energy to unwind and also recover through the night.

The majority of people with an appropriate and balanced level of brainwaves that have sufficient mental security throughout the day are able to block out parts of their minds. As the night gets longer it is likely that the mind will be able to relax and then rest. This is that makes it harder to complete any task at night. Studies have revealed that the process of the mind can change throughout the day, and frequently it can cause a severe form of anxiety. This is because the brain waves are erratic and don't slow down because of the immense stress throughout the daytime. Every thing a person endured during that day is remembered during the night.

The Mind and Also The Brainwaves.

In terms of the mind and how brainwaves react to sleep disorders There are three distinct studies that show how the brain reacts throughout the night. It's been proven that the brain's ability to comprehend and memory processing affects a person's sleep. The more you go out during the daytime more thoughts and memories are likely to be refined by your mind during the night.

Dreams are a result of one's ideas and experiences in real life. The more experiences you have through life as a person, the more you will dream in the night. The capacity to experience more diverse dreams helps the mind relax and create vague thoughts that increase your understanding of your unconscious thoughts in addition to the kind of experiences you've had.

Day vs. Evening.

What's happening inside the brain of people who sleep? The brain of insomniacs is more active at night and struggles to get to the state of calm and relaxation. Within the study of the brain waves during sleep disorders, scientists have found that nerve cells in the mind of those who sleep are more active in the evening. Insomniacs are often prone to having many thoughts going through their heads which lead to sleep disorders. They're constantly in a state of data processing all day long without having the ability of stopping it. In the end, they'll experience difficulties sleeping as well as confront the negative consequences of not getting enough sleep.

The experts say that sleep problems should not be considered as a condition that occurs at night. It's more of an all-day brain disease that makes the brain active throughout the day. Sleep plays an important function in processing and storing memories. Sleep deprivation can affect your memory over the long term. One group got an entire night of sleep, while the other group didn't get much sleep prior to the night before.

The myths.

It's surprising to find that some people believe that they maintain the same level of attention throughout the day. Even though the brain is more active at night than it is in the daytime, it does not mean that the brain can perform at its highest levels.

Focus is not always clear is a result of a study that reveals that insomnia sufferers have higher levels of brain plasticity. The study of what exactly plasticity means and what contributes to the symptoms of sleep problems is not yet clear. What we can say is that ability to change of the brain develops throughout the course of a person's life and is a contributor to various kinds of illnesses in the future. Mind plasticity refers to the ability of the mind to change functionally as well as structurally as a result of physical or environmental factors. Brain plasticity allows us to absorb new information, to learn new things, and continues to develop throughout.

If you experience insomnia, it destroys the brain cells and can lead to the development of brain plasticity. It's more difficult to maintain all levels of memory and concentration as you get older.

The Mind of the Uneasy Mind.

The aim was to find out the possibility that a person who lives stress-related lifestyles suffer from insomnia and how their brain reacts to sleep. The result is that the cognition function in the brain does not change regardless of whether they're suffering from insomnia or not. A majority of research shows that the brain of people who are sleepy wanders during the night. They'll likely have difficulty staying focused the next day, they'll have difficulties focusing on their jobs, their research and also in their personal lives.

In simple terms, your brain is likely to find it difficult to perform optimally the following day, and insomnia sufferers have a hard time performing what they do best. A different aspect of the study compared the memory. The capability to finish any kind of work given to people who are sleepy and to those who had enough rest.

Studies have shown that those who suffer from insomnia cannot recall the majority of their memories throughout the daytime. When it comes to making breakfast, those who are sleeping an adequate amount of sleep head into the kitchen to make snap decisions to start their day.

The brain is trying to keep awake, but it doesn't be able to handle all the information. The brain will become exhausted when you're suffering from insomnia.

The Noodle.

The third and final scientific research focuses on the function of the gray matter in the brain. When people who are insomniacs do not get enough rest at late at night, they'll have an increase of gray matter. If they're suffering with insomnia or are having difficulty sleeping at all, they'll begin to show signs that are related to trauma or depression over time.

The most important thing to be aware of is getting enough food and rest every night. Whatever it takes is to achieve a balanced it is crucial to be able to maintain a high degree of concentration throughout the day to make the most the day.

Concerning your mind, and the way brainwaves react to the stages of sleepiness There are three studies that show how the brain responds to the night. The more you are educated throughout each day time, the greater information and thoughts are processed by the brain in the night.

The brain may be not as active in the night as in the morning does not mean that the brain is able to function at its peak level.

The brain's plasticity is the capacity that the brain has to adapt functionally and structurally according to physical or environmental triggers. In the case of sleepiness, it destroys the brain cells, which leads to the brain's plasticity.

Chapter 3: Sleep Deprived

The body and mind both
It is essential to rest to be productive the following day. If there isn't enough sleep, the gray matter, memory as well as the fancy activities that the brain performs will fall away and insomniacs will have a difficult getting to get through the day. Their minds will definitely wander, and they'll struggle to remain in the present.

The 5 things you should do Everyday
Here's a quick exercise first, take a moment to reflect on the activities you took part in when you woke up this morning. Review the first five things you did. It is possible to turn off the alarm alarm, check the phone or stand, turn on the lights and walk into the bathroom. Whatever your routine is you usually perform all of your routine tasks precisely. It's true that you do of these tasks without having any thought, simply because it became your daily routine.
When you're tired and insomnia, you're not as

focused as you usually are. Your mind may think in the same way it usually does, however it doesn't have all the resources and power required to perform its task effectively. In other terms, you might find it challenging to finish the first five tasks you have to complete in the early morninghours, as well as struggle to complete every task.

If you notice that the task took longer than it ought to in order to complete these tasks it is easy to identify the issue is. If you didn't get enough rest, those five tasks that are meant to take 2 minutes to complete could take longer than 10 minutes. It is possible that you fail to remember to complete something or complete more. It is possible that you do not shut off your alarm or not remember to check your phone for updates. There are many things that can happen but this is just the beginning of the problem when you're suffering from insomnia.

DISRUPTION OF YOUR WORK LIFE

If you are the first night to experience insomnia, you may notice an increase in the level of energy. You may notice that it's difficult to plan your dayor be unable to recall all the details throughout the day.

Your day could begin by waking up, getting dressed to go out, or take a trip to the shops afterwards. Every job requires the fullest concentration to ensure top performance as well as efficiency. Otherwise, you could be a victim of your boss. No matter how exhausted you be, there is only a certain number of days you'll receive a hug from your manager. There are a limited number of sick days that you can use throughout the year. Don't let sleep problems to ruin your professional and personal life. All-in-all you must take control and rid yourself of it.

No matter if you're in the charge for packing the boxes research and writing, must to be on highest level of performance almost every day. The lack of sleep at night could result in a lower performance in the following day.

ARE YOU EXPERIENCING Sleep Starvation?
Each person has their own unique sleep pattern, and experts recommend sleeping 6-8 hours every day. The exact amount depends on the person. Some of us need an extra night of

rest and some require less. At the time of day, losing a few hours of sleep is far more beneficial than sleeping through the night without sleep. For instance instead of acquiring

The loss of two hours of sleep could make you tired however, chances are you'll be capable of completing the task and get everything completed by the end of the day. You'll spend the day battling with basic tasks.

If, for instance, your boss puts a calendar on your desk at work you are able to review the information without difficulty. Understanding the significance of every item in the schedule refers to is the tough part for people who suffer from insomnia. What may appear to be a simple stroll in the park could appear to be a shambles for people suffering from insomnia. Most of the time you lose your concentration and motivation during the day when you aren't getting enough sleep. You'll be looking for the quickest method to get through the day, instead of contemplating the best method to make it through the day.

Although this may not seem likely to you, but it is important to remember that the likelihood of it happening is likely. The effects of insomnia can be a burden to our lives that could cause problems in their work environment, however, it can also affect their private life.

DESTRUCTIONS TO YOUR PERSONAL LIFE
When you look at your own life, consider all that matter to you, things you cherish in your heart. Think about your husband, spouse or children, pet dogs or other aspects. Many people also think of their garden or the transformation project that they've had to complete.

It's your life and the secret to success in your own life is to keep a healthy equilibrium. The majority of people go about their day-to-day routines without giving too much effort into their routine.

easy tasks like preparing a the breakfast meal for your kids taking them to school, getting in the car for a trip for a meal.

Most of the time, these aren't challenging tasks, however insomniacs might be a bit different. When a person's personal life begins to drift out of equilibrium, it triggers uncomfortable moments and they begin to question whether there's a way to restore their normal condition.

It

It doesn't matter if it is due to not having your groceries on time or waking up late, a small amount of stress could build into something beyond control. Sleep issues can cause a significant amount of stress and exhaustion. There will be no type of specific thought within their minds The mind of the person will wander off with random thoughts, without any context. This can be utilized in their professional life. If you're suffering from sleep disorders and you have to prepare your kids to go off to college, then you could not have lunch and forget to iron their clothing, and then the checklist will take place.

Be sure to always put yourself first, as "Vanity is not Egocentric". If you keep putting yourself at the bottom you'll end up in a downward spiral of life, unable to fulfill your ultimate goal in your life.

This is the perfect time to take the lid off a major myth that is prevalent in our society: that of putting yourself first is self-centered, egocentric and selfish. What they don't understand is that if your life is occupied with satisfying the demands of others and not

22

meeting your goals in life You'd be unhappy and destined to fail.

If you live in the home there is a need to maintain your house by walking or cutting grass around the house to search for signs of insects. Whatever you decide to do it is important to remember the steps to complete each task correctly. If you're struggling with insomnia, you will definitely not be able to keep track of things likely, and you'll struggle to get the job completed.

Another important aspect of your life is the relationship you have with your family and friends. If you aren't paying the attention you should give to your spouse because you weren't getting enough rest or sleep, you should expect your relationship to turn to the side.

Controlling Sleepiness

It is difficult to sleep in the absence of any energy left in you. It's easy to feel exhausted and not pay attention to the things going on around you. Your mind is bound to wander often, and your thoughts aren't making any sense. The world is already difficult enough. Consider adding the fact that you're not receiving any kind of rest and must be prepared for every challenge that life throws at you. What do you feel? Bewildered? Worried? You could end up wasting time in your workplace. It is possible that you do not prepare your meals for the family and also upset your children. You may begin to ignore the small things that you normally provide to your lovely relationship. A lot of areas within your life can turn downwards due to insomnia. With these thoughts in mind, now is the right time to prevent your self from falling asleep and have a good night's rest every night. Insomnia, memory loss and insomnia also causes fatigue, irritability and a lack of energy the following day. The body and the mind require rest to function at a high level the next day. If there isn't enough rest, the gray matter memory, memory, and complex tasks of the mind will deteriorate and insomniacs will have a hard to get to the end of their day. Their minds will wander, and they'll have to fight to stay on track throughout the day.

You'd be trying to find the fastest method to get through your day, rather than contemplating the best method to make it through the day.

Chapter 4: The Cure

This is a crucial aspect.

for health and wellness. We need rest to allow our bodies to refuel and recuperate from the day's work. A lot of people struggle with getting to sleep or don't get enough rest and that is where sleep disorders solutions can help.

When it comes to sleeplessness Remedies there are two basic categories.

1. Man-made Solution

The manufactured solution typically sets the price at a high but it typically delivers rapid results. The majority of medications available nowadays are toxic, stuffed with harmful chemicals and cannot be consumed for long periods of time.

2. All-natural Treatment.

Another type of treatment is known as All-natural Solution. This treatment utilizes the body's natural recovery process to overcome sleep disorders.

Whatever type of treatment you choose The goal is to help you fall to sleep and stay in bed. These methods are designed to help you get an additional amount of rest at night.

Eszopiclone, also referred to as Lunesta is a collection of drugs that are able to put people to sleep easily and swiftly. The data show that Lunesta can force people to sleep for 7to 8 hours. It's an effective combination of medications, so be sure you stay away from it unless you can get a restful night to prevent fatigue.

Ramelteon: This group of drugs functions in different ways. It does not cause harm to users, such as sleepiness, grogginess and so on. The most commonly used medicines to induce rest target those who have the CNS (Central Nervous System) by reducing its capabilities and putting the person in a sleepy state. This remedy is suggested for people who have difficulty falling to sleep.

Certain medications have a lengthy activation period in the human body. In the midst of all the latest tablet for rest, Sonata managed to be fully active in the body for the longest amount of time. If someone is having trouble sleeping, a snooze of Sonata tablet is sure to help the person fall asleep and not feeling sluggish the next day.

The medicines in this group are specifically recommended to people who suffer from difficulty staying asleep. This is a chemical solution to the "light sleepers" who are prone to waking up in the evening because of the small amount of

It works by reducing histamine receptors and thus aiding to maintain your sleep even after you've actually fallen to sleep. Since this medication requires you to sleep for a certain amount of time, don't take Silenor in the event that you're not capable of sleeping for at least 7-8 hours each night.

It can have a long-lasting effect on the body since it stays in the body for a prolonged period. If you've suffered from sleep issues for a long period of period of time, this medication will aid them on getting to complete healing.

It is typically used to treat long-term issues as well as sleepwalking. Since the effect of this medication is relentless you may feel tired and exhausted the following day. Another negative side effect of this medication is that it could result in substance abuse and you could have to rely on this drug to go to sleep or be asleep again in the future.

The Benzodiazepines are found in tablets that rest. Triazolam (Halcion), Alprazolam (Xanax), Temazepam (Restoril) in addition to other.

It is essential to undergo a medical examination before taking any kind of tablet for rest. Visit a doctor to conduct a thorough examination. Consult your physician regularly about adverse effects from any medication prior to deciding what tablets to take. Every medication can cause a variety of negative reactions. These negative effects can include an extreme reaction to a medication, a feeling of frustration or sleepiness for a long time to just a couple of. However certain people would definitely prefer to go with natural remedies instead. There is no need to depend on chemical treatments that have dangerous negative effects, specifically after awakening. Instead, you can use natural remedies to improve your sleep pattern and also put an end to your sleep issues.

1. Go camping

If the lure of the television or the phone keeps you awake all late at night, you should take a trip to the tent for to camp. Make use of this time to relax practice yoga, write, recall the thoughts of your mind, or breathe.

According to numerous studies, people who stay away the use of electronic devices as well as engage in relaxation routines like listening to music or meditating were sleeping for two hours earlier than the average. A further thing to bear in mind the impact of electronic gadgets on sleepiness. The research has shown that human-made lighting can negatively impact the body's clocks.

Bath in the sun's natural light and drift off to sleep when the sun sets. In no time you'll be able to reset your sleeping patterns.

2. Songs Treatment

It has been used in the past to fight sleep disorders. It's a recuperative device which can help ease anxiety and stress that can contribute to poor sleep quality. The main advantage of this technique is that it is simple to use and doesn't cause any negative effects.

A number of studies found that those who listen to music that soothes before bed experienced better sleep quality throughout the night, compared to those who do not. If you're having difficulty falling asleep, this might be the solution.

3. Power Down to Enjoy Much Better Rest

Sleep isn't a toggle switch. It is possible to try turning down to get a better night's sleep. To prepare for sleep, it's essential to let go and relax our thoughts.

If you have a hot shower bath prior to bedtime, it'll cause an increase in body temperature and trigger your body to begin preparing for sleep. When you take a relaxing shower the body temperature will definitely decrease the metabolic processes such as heart rate, breathing and digestive rate. Your body will be able to recognize that it's time to lower and relax. Your body will learn in the sense that music in the evening signifies bedtime, If you're a practice of listening to your favorite music prior to going to bed every evening.

It's all about the way you behave and also conditioning. You should take at least one-half hour of wind-down time before bedtime to exercise your breathing or do a leisure exercises to relax your thoughts. The goal of this time of power down is to let your mind know that it's time to relax and sleep, as well as relax.

4. Relax in a Beautiful Area

People who have difficulty sleeping usually have a higher core body temperature immediately before they go to bed in comparison to their more healthy counterparts. This group of insomniacs needs to be patient for a minimum of two to four hours before their body temperature levels begin to decrease and they fall off the rest.

The results of a study show that the ideal temperature for resting is between 16 and 20 degrees Celsius. The brain appreciates cold temperatures while you're trying to fall asleep. A cold, slumbering bedroom can also aid in preventing aging. It aids in the launching of anti-aging hormones known as melatonin. an anti-oxidant with a potent effect that helps with swelling, strengthens the immune system in the body and protects from cognitive damage, as well as cancerous cells.

I could keep going on about the benefits of sleeping well in a cold and chilly environment. The most important factor to increase the production of hormones that fight aging within your body is sufficient sleep.

The initial step is to create the ideal sleeping space by lowering the temperature of your bedroom. Lack of sleep can cause a range of negative effects on the physical and mental health of your sleeping habits are also a risk. You could begin by creating an optimal relaxation environment.

5. Perspire

It's not a secret that exercising improves your sleep and overall well-being. Researchers have found the women who train at moderate intensity for minimum 30 minutes every morning, seven every day of the week, experience less difficulty sleeping than those who exercise less .

Later during later in the later on in the. Morning workouts appear to positively affect our body's rhythms, which results in a boost to our sleep top quality.

One reason that this connection between exercise and sleep could be the body's temperature. This is because lower body temperatures are linked to better sleeping.

Be serious about it, and look for the assistance from a functional medicine specialist If you're struggling to keep your sleeping patterns under control. After you've restart your body clock, and then fall back into your regular rhythm of sleep then you'll begin to reap the benefits of a restful and restorative sleeping.

Sleep is essential for our body to recover and replenish from the stress of our daily lives. The most important factor to increase the production of hormones that fight aging within your body is having sufficient rest.

One reason for this interaction between sleep and exercise could be the body's temperature. The reason is that cooler body temperatures are linked to more restful sleep. When you reset your biological clock, and fall back into your normal rhythm of your sleep and you'll be able to enjoy the benefits of a restful and restorative sleeping.

Chapter 5: Lifestyle Modification

In the previous chapter
We discussed the two primary types of
solutions for getting over sleeping issues. But,
these external influences could not be able to
address the cause of insomnia. You may feel
better after you try these solutions but
insomnia will be completely healed if the
source of the problem is eradicated. If not,
there's the possibility of sleep disorders to
return.
What is the cause of sleep issues? In many
cases, the primary reason for sleep issues is a
poor lifestyle and routines for sleeping. A
simple way to live your life could make a huge
difference to the quality of your sleep.
The cause of insomnia can be triggered by
stress, but it is evident that those who are
constantly stressed are more susceptible to
sleep disorders. When it comes to stressit is.
related sleep disorders, removing anxiety and
stress, or treating insomnia will help. As
discussed in the previous chapter stress and
anxiety affect the quality of sleep, which could

disrupt their sleeping pattern. Therefore, one may struggle to get to sleep at night and stay awake during the day.

It is essential to handle all aspects that you are in an efficient way to ensure you're in a healthy equilibrium. It is crucial to ensure that you get enough rest every day. Sleep is a key element for your physical health.

Insufficient sleep for a brief duration could make you unhappy and unhappy. The long-term effects can be severe such as depression, heart problems and heart attack, stroke to mention some.

According to sleep experts numerous research studies have shown that when people have adequate sleep, they'll not just feel healthier however, they will also boost their chances for living longer, more healthy and also more fulfilled lives.

To avoid insomnia, it is best to steer free of substances like nicotine, alcohol, and the high concentrations of caffeine. Each of these can cause your mind to be constantly stressed. A constant intake of caffeine is sure to cause the mind to become more active than.

Many people require energy to begin their day

and so they choose an to take an energizer. Caffeine is one of the most well-known choices of stimulants to guarantee alertness and also arousal in the early morning hours and throughout the day. However, they aren't aware of the fact that excessive levels of caffeine are only one of the main causes of sleep disorders. It can disrupt the natural balance of wakefulness and sleep.

In this way, those who are insomniacs must stay clear of the drinks that can cause insomnia to ensure the best quality sleep. Do not take a coffee break, and instead grab an ice-cold glass instead and this could be the reason you're having difficulty dropping and staying asleep through the late at night.

Since the body needs regularity, it needs to be at the same time each night and also waking up at exactly at the same time each and every day early in the morning. The body is a fan of a routine. It thrives when it is routine. When you stick to a routine of routine of bedtime and waking time your body is likely to be in a good place. If you can, steer away from rotating routines or late-night celebrations graveyard shifts, or other activities that could disrupt your sleep routine.

If you're having a difficult falling asleep Try drinking and a glass of milk that is cozy. It's a common treatment for insomnia, and it's been proven that it could help you in getting a better night's sleep. In addition, milk helps keep hunger from disrupting your sleep, but it also contains an amino acid known as tryptophan that is converted by the brain into the "relaxing" chemical known as serotonin. Calcium is a powerful metabolic stimulant which reduces anxiety and stress and also reducing levels of the hormone parathyroid that is identified as a factor in insomnia.

In addition it is possible to alter your personal schedule to incorporate periods of yoga or contemplation. There's plenty of evidence to show that yoga and reflection improve sleeping patterns, usually significantly. A time of relaxation to yourself is essential. These techniques can be performed at home, for convenience and privacy. It helps increase the flexibility of your body, ease your mind and relax your body. Try to dedicate at least 30 minutes per day in yoga or meditate. Generally speaking, meditation and yoga exercises are best done early in the morning at a calm area, and in the sun.

To reflect For reflection, all you have to do is to take an incline and then clear your thoughts. Try to focus on the music as it winds down to help slow your body. Once you get used to the idea of doing daily meditation, your mind will relax more quickly in the evening , and you'll have a significantly more easy time going to sleep.

In the first phase we talked about the two primary types of treatments to eliminate sleep issues. Sure, you will be more relaxed after trying the remedies however sleep-related issues are only cured by ensuring that the root of the problem is eradicated. Many people find that the primary cause of sleep issues is having a bad manner of life and sleep routines. Setting up an effective sleep routine yourself is among the most effective self-help methods for sleeping problems. It's a common treatment for insomnia and it's been proven that it could help you in getting better sleep.

Chapter 6: Battling Insomnia

Sleeping problems

It's a long and difficult climb. You're trying to keep your mind from becoming active at night as you attempt to manage sleep issues. If all is going to end, there's no reason to be scared of staying up for a few nights in a row, and then you are.

Stressing can lead to sleepless nights. Get rid of the sleep issues in your mind! All you have to do is to 'turn off' your mind's whirlwind.

In the evening, you want your mind to relax until you're able to easily fall into a deep sleep. A good amount of sleep will help you stay sharp for the next day.

For many busy grownups their only chance to look back at their lives is when they go to the bed! In most cases are the most infamous mistake that stops you from falling to sleep.

If you're one of those who would like to reflect on their lives consider rising earlier so that you get up early in the morning to reflect or even schedule some time at night to create a reflection.

Active EVENING = NEGATIVE Rest

Another reason people do not want to change their routines is because they are juggling multiple things to do in the evening which can be too stimulating, causing them to stay awake instead of feeling tired. Many also like to consume excessive amounts of caffeine in the late at night! Beware of tasks that require you to believe, and require physical effort at night.

Do not miss an extra Night of Rest

Another trick to fall asleep is to plan your sleep. Following training sessions, your brain will definitely be taught to turn off the lights when your clock hits the normal hour for falling asleep.

A regular rest schedule is the most effective way to ensure more restful and high quality sleep. Our bodies develop with regular rest and regularity. There's no universal option. Having a regular routine of rest will definitely help in the fight against sleeplessness that is persistent.

How to turn off"In The Evening

The initial thing do when you've had a meal and cleaned down for the night is to turn off all your electronic devices. Once you're all prepared to sleep, it can increase your focus and it could make it difficult to sleep with your smartphone or computer turned off. Confirm that your digital devices have become habit-forming and you'll never know when it is time to stop.

The light can definitely disrupt your sleeping pattern and make you stay awake. It is advised to not use devices at all costs for at least an hour prior to bedtime.

The idea of catching up before bed is good, but it's not with your electronic gadgets. A physical book as a way to relax prior to going to bed will assist you in getting yourself ready for bed. It is suggested to read in a different area since you don't want you to become occupied within the space you'll need to sleep in.

The songs can help in relaxing your mind, and take your anxiety and stress. Attention to anything interesting or loud is sure to stimulate the mind, and it'll be more difficult to fall into a deep sleep.

Another suggestion is to plan your day before you go to bed. Making notes of ideas for the next day can help to clear your mind.

Staying awake at night while constantly telling

yourself that you need to keep in mind something is sure to keep your mind occupied. It will help in calming down and fall asleep faster.

Another thing you can try is having an enjoyable drink like tea prior to going to getting to bed. You must stay clear of high amounts of alcohol, caffeine, and drinks that contain lots of sugar. The perfect drink is one that can help calm your mind and body and help your body relax.

It is a time to relax and unwind. If you don't find pleasure in drinking tea, then consider having a small snack prior to going to going to bed. It doesn't matter, a small dessert is a good idea because sometimes, the reason for having trouble sleeping is simply due to hunger.

Another way to ensure certain that you are resting comfortably is to reduce your room's temperature. The best way to achieve this is to set the thermostat of your room to be just a little cooler. The body is programmed in a way so that when it is in an environment that is cooler it will definitely receive an indication that it's time for a rest.

It is a good idea to take a short shower before getting ready for bed. Ideally , a refreshing shower will quickly cool. If you prefer, you could consider acquiring the bed follower or a cooler cushion or take a short walk prior to the bed.

Each one of the essential items listed above could be part of your bedtime routine. Try to test them out and note down which ones work best for you, and your schedule. In any case you won't have any difficulty falling asleep or staying in bed for the next time.

If you're trying to get rid of sleep issues it is actually trying to prevent your mind from becoming active in the night. There's no reason to be worried about staying up all night in a row, as well as wondering when you will ever be over.

When you go to bed, you would like your mind to relax until you are able to fall asleep quickly. A good amount of sleep helps you stay sharp for the next day and gives you a restful night's sleep.

Another reason people fail to sleep off is the fact that they have numerous tasks to complete at night which are too stimulating, causing the impression of feeling tired.

Chapter 7: How to get the best rest every night

How to Get a Great
Night's Rest ... All Night
The most aggravating aspect of a good rest is it may be difficult to discern. There are numerous things that could affect the quality of our sleep, and could cause us to continue on the downward slope, far from the holy grail that is 8 uninterrupted hours of restorative, deep sleep. The main issue, and the reason for this is, how can we ensure better quality sleep? The answer, thankfully is much simpler than you might think.

If you're in search of an easy-to-follow list of steps to help support healthy sleep habits, our twelve tips for healthy sleep is an ideal starting point.

1--Set aside time for rest.

Routine is the mother of a good night's sleep. One of the most important aspects to creating an effective sleep routine is understanding the body's clock. Simply put What is your ideal sleep-wake cycle? Do you prefer to be an early-bird or an or a night owl? It is possible to move it forward or backwards according to your needs until you find the perfect point of a schedule that is in harmony with your life and requires perfection when you find it.

It's a routine that's best for the most optimal results most likely to follow strictly. This means waking up and going to bed at the exact time every day, excluding weekends off. Constantly changing the time you sleep and wake along with the set hours of sleep will take you to nowhere other than Frustrationville.

2--BE ENERGETIC

It is the reason for an excellent night's rest that you're aware of. Perhaps you are also the most scared by too. Exercise means better rest. Since exercise increases your body's temperature, the subsequent reduction in temperature can promote sleep, which is a result of the feeling of being sleepy. In the same way, exercise helps remove sleep-related disorders like anxiety and stress, depression symptoms, and anxiety.

When you plan your activities to start your day you should factor in an exercise session that will raise the heart rate, intensify the effort of breathing and cause you to be slightly sweaty. The more vigorously you choose to exercise and the more positively your sleep quality will definitely be affected.

However, a short walk in the morning is enough to improve your sleep quality, however don't anticipate miracles to happen over night. The commitment to regular rest will reap benefits after a couple of months. Simply hold your horses.

Pro-tip: Make sure to complete your workout about 3 hours before the time you go to bed. This is due to the fact that exercise can speed up your metabolism increases your body temperature, and encourages the release of cortisol (one of the hormones that increase the level of awareness).

3--Light exposure

One important aspect that can affect our circadian rhythms is sunlight. From a transformational perspective the human body is not built to take in the wealth of artificial light that we've come to expect in the last century. The cycle of your sleep and wake is, generally controlled by melatonin (the sleep-inducing hormone) that circulates through your body. If it's dim, the brain releases more of it, which makes you feel more ready for sleep, while it releases lesser when it's bright, making you noticeably more alert.

Naturally, adding artificial light in this mix (e.g. televisions and digital screens as well as, as infamously mobile phones) can be enough to disrupt this natural process. What can you do to assist in restoring the balance in your body? Here's an easy to read checklist of 8 items to take care of and beware of ...:.

Do expose yourself to bright sunlight as early in the morning as is possible. This will aid in managing the natural electrical system that controls your sleep and can also assist in waking you up with a more natural manner.

Do your best to stay outdoors during the day for as long as you can.

Keep your curtains up and also let the sun shine in your home throughout the day.

Use an light treatment box in case getting enough natural light is difficult (i.e. in winter, especially if you reside in a place that gets less normal hours of sunlight).

Do not take your phone to the bed and keep

scrolling.

If you're required to wake up to take a shower break make sure you don't turn the lighting on in the middle of the night.

Don't sleep in a room that is light - attempt to block any light in your sleeping environment during your go to bed.

Do not fall asleep fast after watching television or doing a computer work - because, as when using a mobile phone the light that is emitted by screens reduces the release of Melatonin.

4--DIET REGIMEN.

This is a significant one, and it is a good reason to do so. The food and drinks that you consume throughout the day have significant effects on the quality of your sleeping. But, despite the benefits of a healthy diet being healthy, achieving it is an absolute cake-walk.

To assist you in a positive way, your overall experience is of top quality:

High levels of caffeine remain in the system for about 12 hours and pure nicotine could also trigger your ability to drift into a deep sleep.

Alcohol with a restriction - contrary to what is commonly believed alcohol can make you feel sleepy but it can also reduce the body's ability to go into the deeper sleep stages.

Take it easy with the fluids before bed A bladder that is full needs clearing sooner ...

If you are unable to eliminate these foods from your in full, you can reduce the amount of sugar as well as the carbohydrates you consume throughout the day.

5--Reflection.

It's not necessarily a matter of ripping out your yoga pants, and putting on the Spotify mix of Tibetan singing or whale tracks and also focusing on the flow of blood flowing through your body while expressing gratitude for the sunshine. Yes, this kind of meditation is great however it might not suit your needs. Think of meditation as a time of quiet and a time to focus on your own way to address the concerns or worries you have. There's nothing wrong with carrying around such thoughts. It's just human, but there are incredibly effective ways to deal with them.

Many people prefer to meditate through music and extend with different methods to concentrate their minds on specific areas of the body. There's a meditation routine for all kinds of minds and a quick internet search can provide you with an abundance of meditation ideas.

It's very simple to use breathing exercise that can help you relax a bit more:

Dress the same way you normally for bed. Then you enter, lie on your back and shut your eyes.

Apply your left hand to your upper body and ease your abdomen to the point of relaxation.

Breathe via your nose. allowing your lungs fully and noting the hand that expands (hint that it's the left hand).

Breathe in through your nose and press as much air as you can, and as hard as possible.

What is the method the right-hander of yours moving at present?

Repeat the process, and note precisely how your level of relaxation improves with each exhale-inhale.

6--Optimise your sleep setting.

This may be the most neglected element of the problem. A well-designed sleeping environment can be limited to a few qualities:

Dark.

Cool (ideally between 18 and 20 levels Celsius).

Well is aerated.

Quiet.

Comfy.

The schedule is designed for intimacy and rest only.

Everything taken into account It's a very important tiny list. How exactly these things can be completed, or just the amount you'd like to become in creating this kind of space is completely up to you. But if you apply the six basic elements what else will be the common garnish.

Routine is the basis of a good night's sleep. A key element of creating an effective sleep routine is to understand the rhythm of your day. Continuously changing the time you go to bed and awake, and the hours you are supposed to be sleeping will result in nothing other than frustrationville.

Exercise = better sleep.

The food and beverages you drink throughout the day have significant influence on how you sleep.

Chapter 8: Benefits of a good night's sleep

We have a good night's sleep can bring about several positive results. Good rest is the only way to bring good results.

Here are 9 of the most significant benefits that a good night's sleep will provide:

Lower risk of stroke, Alzheimer's disease as well as cardiovascular diseases

The pounding heartbeat it is not uncommon to experience upon waking after only an hour of sleep? The rise in your heart rate in long-term periods of insufficient rest enough to raise your blood pressure that, if untreated, will not only increase the risk of developing heart disease, but also for strokes and Alzheimer's too.

Focused and improved performance

The mind needs rest just like the body. If the mind is rid of the harmful chemicals that build up during the day, then rest is. A good night's rest is the mind is clean!

This means that while you'll be feeling a lot more energetic after a good, restful sleeping, you'll also be more prepared to focus and focus more effectively during the course of your day.

A lack of sleep increases the chance of weight increase

This is due to the effects of deprival at rest on the two hormones that regulate your cravings Leptin and the hormone ghrelin. Leptin reduces hunger, and Ghrelin increases it. Do you have a guess as to which is the most effective after an evening of sleepiness ...

The risk of establishing Type 2 Diabetic issues

In direct connection with the previous reduction in leptin levels as well as the increase in ghrelin likely lead you to consume excessively as well as consume a lot of the food you normally desire - possibly ones that are high in sugar and refined carbohydrates. A prolonged consumption of both for a long period of time can increase your chances of developing Kind 2 diabetic issues.

A man is sitting on a patio and also yawning. The effectiveness of your sports will surely be raised.

Studies have revealed that the quality of sleep positively impacts the efficiency of sports across the range of technical abilities including speed, response time, and accuracy. These research studies have also revealed a strong connection between good rest and greater psychological well-being.

Other research studies have also linked low quality of rest to an enlargement of physical capacity outside of the circle of athleticism. In a study that included nearly three hundred older women, who had a median aged that was 83.5 years, the results showed that limited and inadequate rest caused slower walking rates, lower grip strength, and an higher difficulty in performing basic exercises on their own.

Better immune features

Absolutely, a good night's sleep helps to boost the strength of your body immune system that is more well-equipped to help stop the progression of colds.

A well-known study proved this by depriving the anxious people of rest and then squirting the cold virus directly in the noses. The study was conducted for two weeks, the study showed that those who slept less than 7 hours per night were 3 times more likely to catch cold than those who were resting for eight hours.

The Pro Pointer is 8 hours of sleep has been found to increase your body's capability to fight and fight off the rhinitis that is acute.

Good sleep can have an enormous impact on your emotions and mood. A rejuvenating sleep and because of it, a continuous high-quality sleep will surely help to maintain your positive mood. How often have you experienced a restful night and then woken with a bad mood? It also assists in lubricating your social interactions, which together with a greater ability to be able to pay attention and draw attention to yourself, will yield a positive outcome. You'll also be able to register the impressions that others express.

In simple terms, getting victimized can lead to lower or less social skills, increased negative emotions, as well as a less ability to recognize the psychological signals of others.

A lot less swelling

The body's swelling is a defense mechanism. It occurs when an object of international origin such as a microorganism, fragment or something that is in between, enters the body. In many cases, the body misinterprets its cell or tissues as being international which could lead to more extensive various issues that can be characterized as type 1 diabetes mellitus as well as an autoimmune disorder.

Better rest health and wellbeing can help reduce the risk of swelling that is persistent.

Better memory retention.

In the rest of your day, among the activities that take place within your brain is assessment and also organization of your memories. For those who are in the short-term memory banks are arranged and then transferred into long-term storage.

Maybe you've also noticed that when you're exhausted, it's harder to recall particular details? A better, more consistent rest will assist you in avoiding these memory gaps.

The rise in the heart rate during prolonged periods of sleep deprivation can increase the blood stress that relaxes you. This is left untreated will increase the risk of developing heart diseases, but for strokes and Alzheimer's too.

The mind demands rest as easily as the body needs rest. It is during this time that the mind is cleansing its body of the toxins that are usually accumulate during the day. A good night's rest results in the mind is clean!

Chapter 9: Insufficient eating and drinking Consumption can cause insomnia.

Food intake prior to bed can affect our sleep
A large amount of food consumed prior to
going to bed could affect the way we sleep. It is
important to determine when you will take
your meals in the evening. Don't eat anything
during the night as it could affect your sleep
cycle.
Medical Health
There are certain conditions that can be
associated with insomnia, such as the diabetes
condition, Alzheimer disease, chronic pain,
cancers, asthma cardiovascular disease
Parkinson illness, thyroid overactivity. If you are
concerned about any health problem, it's
important to consult a medical professional to
see if your doctor can help you.
Alcohol and Caffeine Consumption
Consuming alcohol or caffeine could affect our
sleep because they're stimulants, which could
influence your sleep. You need to limit the
consumption of alcohol and caffeine so that you
can be able to sleep comfortably.

Chapter 10: The effects of medication, mental health and work Schedule can cause insomnia.

Mental Health Problem

Problems with anxiety can affect our mental health, and can influence our sleep patterns. Individuals struggling with depression might disturb their sleep because of anxiety and mental illness. One of the most important things in being patient is to be patient, no what the issue you must remain patient and believe in your abilities and seek out help to over come it.

There is no need to be embarrassed, you may seek assistance from loved ones or your health professional They will be happy to help. If you are suffering from mental illness, are suffering from is a good reason to seek assistance.

MEDICATION

The kind of medication we be taken can impact our sleep. These medications contain stimulants which can disrupt the sleep cycle.

Work Schedule

The nature of the job may be a contributing factor to an individual to experience sleepiness.

There was a time when in which I had an assignment that was not too demanding. With this kind of job is in a position of freedom and you know many guidelines, and I could sleep well.

I have a new job which requires me to be at a certain time, and close by with no time off and this impacted my sleeping patterns. Your work could affect your sleep. ensure that you schedule your time correctly so that you are able to relax and enjoy your sleep.

People who are older tend to experience insomnia because of a change in their sleeping patterns. People who are older tend to fall asleep earlier in the evening and get up earlier. The older people are less active and they're more likely to rest, which could impact their sleep at night.

As people age, they are more likely to experience issues with their health, which could affect their sleep patterns in the night. Additionally, the use of prescription medications can influence their sleep.

Chapter 11: Risk factors and symptoms of insomnia

INSOMNIA is a condition that can affect an individual at any time IN the future. The symptoms of INSOMNIA is listed below.
* Depression, anxiety and Irritation
* It becomes difficult to fall asleep.
* Waking up in the middle of sleep
* It's difficult to get back to sleep
* Inability to connect with friends.
* Waking up earlier rather than the time I had planned
* Daytime sleepiness
* The thought of sleepinglessness
* Increase in accidents
* Tiredness

The risk factors for insomnia

Nearly EVERYBODY has a RISK of developing INSOMNIA and the people who are at MOST RISK INCLUDE
Individuals under pressure
A stressful situation could trigger insomnia try as hard as you can reasonably expect to not to

put yourself in a stressful situation and in the event that you're feeling pressured, you may have thought of a strategy to overcome the stress.

Problems with emotional well-being

People who suffer from psychological health problems can trigger Insomnia The first thing you have to do is to find an solutions to your mental health to enable you to be a healthy and happy person.

Ladies

Females are more likely to suffer from sleep disorders due to hormone issues, such as menopausal changes and pregnancy, as well as the menstrual cycle.

Poor Sleeping plan

One of the reasons that cause insomnia is due to a inadequate sleep habits. If you continue to disrupt your sleeping routine, you're likely to cause Insomnia. You must schedule your sleep in a way that is suitable to sleep at a particular time each day and rise at a particular regular time in order that your body is adjusted to it.

Old age

As we grow OLD OUR sleeping pattern may become DISRUPT as a result of illness and

OTHER issues, OLDER PEOPLE ARE AT RISK of INSOMNIA.

INSOMNIA can affect the body IN different ways, including increasing medical conditions like OBESITY and heart diseases and a weak immune system. INFLAMMATION, STROKE, ASTHMA attacks, HIGH BLOOD PRESSURE AND AN INCREASE IN SEIZURES, PAIN, DIABETES MELLITUS.
INSOMNIA can ALSO have an effect on OUR mental health such as anxiety or depression and FRUSTRATION. INSOMNIA is able to ALSO affect OUR life expectations; INSOMNIA CAN SHORTEN OUR life by denying us the kind of life we must leave. The good news is that it is possible to overcome the affliction.

Chapter 12: Lifestyle that encourage Sleep

There are some ways you can take to overcome insomnia. There are certain actions and lifestyles you should focus on to get rid of insomnia. This includes

* Stop worry
* Do not take a nap during the day
* You should go in Bed at a certain time, and then wake up at a certain time
* Avoid the consumption of stimulant and alcohol.
* Do not eat a large meal prior to bed
Do not use your the phone prior to the bed
* Practice Exercise
Always ensure that you get back to bed
• Make sure your bed is cozy

Stop Stressing

Do not use nighttime to think about everything you have to think about doing in the day, and instead make use of night time to rest. Night isn't a time to worry, but to rest, try to sleep as much as you can be expected to rest. Think about if that night was the last one you will not have any worries about.

Do not take a nap during the day.

Avoid sleeping in the daytime; it will not help

you get sleeping at night. Try as much as you can reasonable be expected in order to end your taking a nap in the day. sleeping in can affect the way you sleep in the evening.

You should go to bed at a particular time and then wake up at a certain time.
Try to sleep every day at the same time and get early at the same times each day. This will assist you in regulate your sleep pattern and allow you feel great rest throughout the night, once your body is accustomed to it. The time you sleep at every day affects the rhythm of your sleep. It is important to create a schedule that can help you establish a regular sleeping pattern.
Stop the sale of alcohol and stimulants
Do not drink alcohol, nicotine or caffeine late at night as they can affect the quality of your sleep. If you have to conquer sleep disorders, try as the amount that is believed to reduce the intake of caffeine, alcohol and nicotine, particularly at the end of the evening and at night, as the stimulant can greatly affect your sleep.

Avoid eating large meals prior to going to bed
Don't eat a large meal prior to going to bed at
night. there are some who like to eat late at
late at night, and this could affect the quality of
your sleep. do your best to to eat dinner in the
evening. Don't eat meals before the time of bed
because it can affect the quality of sleep.
Do not use your phones before the bed
Beware of mobile phones prior to bedtime as
they emit blue light to your body , which can
disrupt our sleep. If you use your phone at
night, it can make it difficult to fall asleep and
can cause you feel awake at evening. Take
every precaution to not use your phone and
computer at bedtime. Find a program that can
assist you decrease the intensity of blue light
getting into your eyes at night time since blue
light can disturb the sleep cycle.
Practice Exercise
Try to engage in exercise throughout the day,
and it will allow you to rest comfortably at
night. Do whatever it takes to avoid doing
exercise before bedtime since this will keep you
awake and not induce sleep.

Always ensure that you go back to bed

If you wake up in the middle of the night , go back to bed and keep an idea in top of your mind that you are laying down until you are asleep. With the passage of time, your mind will begin to process the thought and help in sleeping.

You can make your bed comfortable
Making your sleeping ENVIRONMENT more comfortable. When your sleep ENVIRONMENT is comfortable, you will easily fall asleep. The act of reading a book before bed will help you sleep comfortably.

Chapter 13: How to use the Cognitive-Behavioral Treatment to get rid of insomnia

One of the most effective ways strategies to beat insomnia is to concentrate on your thinking. The reason is a fact that someone has trouble sleeping during the night. This can significantly impact our thoughts negatively, and this causes our minds to focused on the negative aspects of sleep.

When I first started experiencing insomnia, it was a bit strange to me , and I was in shocked to discover that I do not go to fall asleep in the same way that I did prior to that. I saw my primary doctor and we discovered that the root of my sleeplessness was due to the usage of computers in the evening and also taking part in some unpleasant activities prior to when I go to bed. The usage of PC as well as the activities were the main reason behind my insomnia. When I was experiencing a sleepless night, I conducted some research and discovered that insomnia is a cause of cancer. This made me worried and made me think , and I went to my primary doctor.

The best way to overcome insomnia is change your mindset the idea that insomnia is an illness that is harmful to health and is overcome by altering our behavior and habits. Do not think of insomnia as something you should be ashamed of Change your negative beliefs which are making you sleepy. The process of overcoming insomnia requires patience, as you alter your habits and lifestyle, you must be patience so that your body can adjust to the new way of life. Do your best to sleep at a certain time and wake up at a particular time. Be aware of thoughts that are making you feel anxious about sleeping Your mind may be telling you that you'll not get a good night's sleep tonight, alter the idea and remind yourself that you'll always rest comfortably. There was a time that I would wake up in the early hours of the morning and I couldn't sleep until the next morning. This was very disappointing and I began to worry about it. The way to deal with this issue was confess that I sleep in a stupendous way whenever I wake up in the mid-night in order to get back to sleep. It is important to take care of your life style What are the actions you need to take care of to rest comfortably. It is advisable to do this, but you should also support it with a positive notions. In order to overcome insomnia, it is essential to be aware of the causes of insomnia so that you can be able to conquer it. Sleepiness can be a result of anxiety about sleeping Don't view insomnia as a negative thing as it's something that is easily conquered.

Do not be depressed just accept that Insomnia isn't a problem and is something that you are able to easily an issue overcome. Just be patient and collaborate with your primary medical doctor to overcome Insomnia. The effects of insomnia can begin to affect your thoughts, such as I am not sleeping tonight try as hard as you can reasonably expect for you to overcome negative thoughts and allow your mind to sleep with the intention to sleep well. It is not necessary to be desperate and want an instant results, but you do must collaborate with your physician to get rid of insomnia.

Chapter 14: Lifestyles that encourage sleep

Use the method that is outlined to get rid of
Insomnia
Sleep Restrictions
One method you can try to conquer insomnia
includes sleep restrictions, the process in which
you stop yourself from sleeping. If, for instance,
you awake in the early hours of the morning
and are finding it difficult to return to sleep.
You can do other things like reading a book. It is
best to try and go back to sleep, however after
a few hours of not getting sleeping, you'll be
able to awake and start to engage in other
activities. This will help you sleep more soundly
the following night. Do your best to not nap
throughout the day to ensure you are able to
rest better in the evening. I would suggest
having a routine including time for sleeping and
the time you wake up.
Recondition your brain
Do whatever can be required to change the way
you think about your brain. Once your mind
know that the evening is for sexual sleep and
sexual sex. Try as hard as you can to change

your brain's programming. One method by to rewire the brain you have is to keep clear of naps during the morning, with the intention that you are able to rest throughout the night. Create a schedule that will aid you in determining when to go to bed and when you will awake.

Relaxation Exercise

Do your best to calm your mind prior to going to bed and also to relax your mind in the time when you awake from your sleep so that you are able to get back to the sleep.

Chapter 15: Medication for insomnia

If you suffer from insomnia, it is advisable to consult your doctor Your doctor will conduct an assessment of your physical, medical state and your history of sleep. Your physician will ask you to record your sleeping patterns over a period of time in order to know what needs to be done.

Acute insomnia that is mild is not a need for treatment. you can beat this kind of insomnia by maintaining a healthy sleep routine. It is essential to collaborate with your physician in order to beat insomnia. There are several medications that can be purchased to treat Insomnia It is recommended to utilize cognitive behavioral therapy and a lifestyle way of life changes to conquer Insomnia. Prescriptions are used for a short duration, and they are employed to temporarily treat insomnia. Prior to you begin medication, it's advised to consult with your physician.

Benzodiazepines

The medicine is used to treat insomnia and the patient may become dependent to it.

Antidepressants

They also aid in the treatment of insomnia and antidepressants such as remeron, the nefazodone and doxepin are helpful in the treatment of insomnia.

Melatonin

It is also beneficial for treating insomnia as we age the body's ability to produce melatonin decreases. That is the reason why melatonin supplements are beneficial for Insomnia treatment, especially for people who are old. Melatonin assists us in falling asleep, and can help us to sleep for a long duration. Ramelteon is commonly utilized for treatment of insomnia.

Non benzodiazepines

Medicines like zaleplon, eszopiclone and zolpidem can be beneficial in the treatment of insomnia.

Drugs that are available over The Counter Drugs

There are many drugs used to treat Insomnia. These medications contain antihistamines that can be effective in the treatment of insomnia.

Chapter 16: Diagnostics and Treatment of Insomnia

We've discussed the causes of insomnia, and explained why it's difficult to treat, so is the time to take action! We assume that you suffer from insomnia or at least you think you could be. If so you must get it under control before it turns into a persistent issue.

What is your initial step?

The first thing to do is need to establish a solid diagnosis.

The First Steps to Diagnose

See your physician and discuss the problem. They will conduct an extensive history. They will also inquire about any issues you are currently experiencing throughout your day. This will allow them to determine whether the problem is a chronic insomnia issue or if it's more long-term, i.e. it's been recurring for a longer time, but isn't related to specific events.

You must definitely check in with your physician for the following reasons:

* If you've experienced problems sleeping for a while and you've attempted to alter your routine, e.g. alter the temperature of the room, take a more relaxed nap and still haven't worked.
* The amount of time that your sleep issue is ongoing is spread over several months
Sleep deprivation has a negative impact on your life and you're having a hard time coping.
difficult to deal with the stress.

These are the red flags that should bring you to the nearest doctor's clinic.

The doctor will try to discover what's the cause of your insomnia, as this is the path to treatment. If your doctor believes that it's your habits and thoughts that are causing the problem, you might be suggested to CBT which is also known as cognitive Behavioural Therapy. It is a type of therapy and counselling that will help you to change your mindset and your thoughts by removing negative thinking patterns and focusing on the ones that will get you to where you want to be, i.e. to sleep!

It is highly likely that your physician is going to prescribe sleeping tablets to you due to the many side effects that can be associated the use of these medications. In the past the pills were the most popular treatment option however, times have changed and we're now more familiar with the best ways to manage sleep issues. Apart from that, sleeping pills are extremely addicting, and it's not unusual to get dependent on these drugs. The only situations where sleeping pills are prescribed are when the insomnia is very serious, or if all alternative treatments have been tried but were unsuccessful.

Another option your doctor may think about is sending you to an insomnia clinic for additional tests. This will allow the doctor determine an accurate explanation for your sleeplessness, and be followed by better guidance regarding how to manage it.

Sleep Evaluation & Sleep Clinics

Your physician may send you to an apnea or sleep clinic. It is a facility that treats sleep disorders including sleep apnoea or insomnia. The reason behind this is because these ailments are extremely difficult to evaluate while people are still awake and they must be asleep for the medical professional to be able look at what's happening and what the severity is.

These kinds of clinics aren't like normal hospital settings, and are designed to appear more like bedrooms or hotels, to aid the patient in falling more quickly to sleep, and allow for the evaluation to be carried out. But, there is still a hospital under the hood and has an abundance of highly-specialized lab equipment to aid in assessing the situation.

It will be suggested to relax and then, obviously, attempt to sleep. You'll be lying in a comfy bed and it's like staying at home however, you'll be connected to various monitoring devices, which analyze the activity of your brain, your movements while you sleep and the speed that your eyes move as well as your heartbeat. If you are suffering from sleep apnoea or snoring it is also checked for more details.

Sleep labs are highly specialised diagnostic instrument for doctors, however they're not widespread and are in a very limited availability. The doctor might recommend a specialist clinic like this, but bear in mind that waiting time for seeing a specialist may be long. It is possible to visit an individual sleep clinic however, you'll need to pay for it and in some cases, the cost could be quite high.

You're likely to be required to keep a journal of your sleeping patterns for a few weeks or even a month prior to your visit to the clinic for sleep. That means you must record the times you fell asleep as well as the time you got up, how long you took to fall asleep, as well as the time you awoke. Also, try to record the time you got up. This will give the staff in the sleep lab with more data to work with and can be compared to the data the sleep lab studies provide when you're there being evaluated.

Medical Treatment for Insomnia

Like all things today there are medical options that you can take to treat insomnia, in addition to self-help and herbal methods. We'll discuss self-help methods and holistic treatments in a future section, but for now, we must focus on the medical treatment options.

You can visit either of the two locations to look seek out medications to treat insomnia - a pharmacist or your physician. Always consult your physician first, as they know your medical history and can examine the issue in a deep manner, as well as checking for potential interactions with medications you're taking.

The kinds of medicines you can use to treat sleeplessness (by prescription) comprise Benzodiazepine-Hypnotics, non-benzodiazepine hypnotics, and a different kind of drug known as Melatonin Receptor Agonist. These medications all contain an element of sedation which is why you must be cautious when operating machines or driving once you've taken some of them. It is likely that you'll be taking it about around an hour prior to going to going to bed. You'll notice that your body is relaxed as does your mind. same, and your sleep is much more easily. These are, in fact, an alternative to a sleeping pill, and you must be very cautious with dosage, and make sure to follow the advice of your physician only.

If you are able to combat your insomnia with no medication, this will always be the most efficient option. The medications for sleep disorders tend to have adverse effects and also the real risk of developing addiction. If you are able to manage the issue by focusing on the whole it is likely be the better choice for you. If you believe you'll need medicine in the near future however, talk to your doctor regarding the best treatment for you.

Non-Medical Treatments for Insomnia

There are many alternatives you can go for when dealing with insomnia, that do not require the use of tablets. We'll discuss herbal and self-help remedies in the near future however there are several mental and physiological training options to explore as well. They've been proven to be highly effective and often are among the first options your physician will recommend to you.

Cognitive Behavioural Therapy (CBT) and Relaxation
The mindset that drives CBT changes your thinking patterns and therefore if you have an uneasy mind-set about sleep, e.g. you are worried about sleeping in the evening because you believe that you're not going to get enough sleep, this creates a cycle of things to happen. CBT can assist you to transform your thoughts into something more positive which can help you go to sleep much more comfortably your evening.

CBT can be a lengthy and sometimes lengthy process and one that requires commitment and faith by the person taking it on. If you're not convinced it's going to work then it's probably not be for you. However, it's worth trying it is important to commit your entire self to it, if you really want it to be successful. You'll work with a qualified counsellor to improve your thinking and will offer you a variety of exercises to do, that are designed to test your thoughts and transform them into positive and productive.

Relaxation training is a different kind of CBT technique and also a stimulation control. We are all too focused before we fall asleep, e.g. we constantly check our phones or watch high action films prior to going to getting to sleep. Being completely relaxed and to be in a state of mind , sleep is more easy is essential. Controlling your stimulation is equally about teaching your brain to know when it's the time to fall asleep, through your surroundings and the way you structure your schedule. It is often enough to relax the body and mind when it is the right time and fix a sleep disorder.

The best thing about CBT and behavioral therapies is that they can learn them your self to some level and practice them at your own home. Of course, you'll require to be taught the fundamentals by a professional firstto make sure you're performing these exercises correctly. Relaxation training could also comprise the concept of progressive muscle relaxation. It helps the person learn to tighten and relax muscle groups creating a sense of peace and tranquility. Breathing exercises and meditation could also prove beneficial and are alternatives that your physician could with. Meditation is something you can do at your home.

Many people have difficulty initially with meditation because they don't believe it can be beneficial for them. It's about giving it trial, but to achieve that it is necessary to take the plunge. Much like CBT generally You must believe it's going to work.

A simple meditation practice is something like this:
* Find a quiet place in a place where you're not likely to be constantly disturbed
* Choose your time before bedtime, as this is the time you'll want to relax as much as you can.
• Turn off your mobile and shut the curtains, ensure that the space is dark and cool/warm exactly as you are at home.

• Be at ease with the place you're sitting or lying. Bring lots of blankets and pillows Make sure you don't end up in a position that is awkward.

Shut your eyes, and focus upon your breathing. Relax your breathing into your nostrils inwards for a number of ten after which you should hold it for five minutes. Inhale slowly out of your mouth for another ten seconds.

Repeat this procedure until you realize that your mind is slowing.

If any thoughts pop into your head, allow them to flow by acknowledging their presence and let them flow into the opposite direction - do not allow them to take up much time

After a brief period you'll notice that your mind has calmed down and your body is a bit heavy This is the state you must be in

Then, shift your focus to your toes and tense your feet, and hold them for five seconds before letting them go.

Repeat this procedure for every major muscle of your body, beginning from your toes' tips and all the way towards the crown of your head. at the time you've finished you'll be at peace and relaxed.

It could take some time to perfect it but that's fine. It is not possible to be able to do it all in the very beginning!

As you will see, there's plenty of assistance on the ready for those suffering from insomnia, and many options for treatment to explore. It's all about finding the appropriate one for you. However, the non-medical and medical options have proven to be highly effective for a lot of sleepers in the past.

Chapter 17: Self-Help and Herbal Remedies to Treat Sleepiness

In our last chapter , we discussed non-medical and medical methods for treating insomnia, as well in the next chapter, we will concentrate more on self-help and herbal treatments that are efficient in their own way.

Naturally, we must take a note of caution when it comes to making a decision to take a herbal remedy under your own. Always consult with your doctor before you start, particularly if are taking other medicines already. They can interact with each other and render your medication completely null and void or even less efficient. It's best to test things out prior to you start. If you're able to see the green light, which is likely to happen in most instances that you will be most welcome to test the various herbal cures for insomnia.

First, let's talk about some of the more standard self-help techniques you could explore. They range from meditation, similar to the one we discussed in the previous chapter and more general subjects that include relaxing before sleeping, having an ice bath, etc. It may seem like easy, but they're extremely efficient!

Let's look at a few right now.

Effective self-help treatments for Insomnia

It's really about an array of rules and guidelines. If you make a change to your sleep habits could result in a significant increase in the severity of your insomnia. This is a great option for insomnia that is chronic, and not for insomnia that is acute, e.g. caused by a particular occasion, which is expected to be gone in a short time. But it doesn't mean that you shouldn't take a shot! Relaxing your mind, you'll be able to forget all your worries and possibly fall asleep more easily.

You can regulate your sleep time
Do your best to fall asleep every night at the same moment each day, and wake up every day at the same time each day. It is recommended to get to bed whenever you are tired and do not attempt to try to force yourself to sleep. By

establishing an established bedtime routine and you'll notice that you will naturally get tired around exactly the same moment. This is a great way to get your body's rhythm back into time, especially when you're in shifts, or on a long-distance trip and ended up in a state of jet lag.

Try pre-bedtime relaxation
In the hours before you go to bed, try to unwind as much as you can. Relax in a warm bath, relax with a book or just relax and try to relax your mind to the maximum extent you can. When you allow yourself to relax your body releases the relax hormone, known as dopamine. This can help you go to sleep easily. Many people enjoy reading books, while others prefer the warm bath. Perhaps add some lavender to your bath or the warm milk.

Beware of stimulation before bed
Beware of anything that puts your senses in high alert. This includes Facebook, checking emails and engaging in any kind of argumentative conversation or reading books that enthral you or watch action movies or

horror films that will keep you on the edge of your seat. You must wind down and not get exhausted!

A lot of us are at risk of keeping our mobiles on the bedside table to be ready in the event that someone calls or a message on Facebook or Twitter comes in. Be careful! Make your phone silent. Be assured that the alarm will not stop!

Create a Sleep-Worthy Environment

Make sure that your bedroom is cozy and well-equipped for a good night's to sleep. Be sure that it's silent, dark and well-ventilated. You don't want to be hot or cold. Set up curtains that are thick to block out light and especially the security lights that are outside. They are known to produce an enormous chink of light in the middle of your bedroom! It is also possible to wear an eye mask, or wear the earplugs.

Do a lot of exercise

It is logical to assume that if you've done a lot of exercising and your body is likely to be exhausted, thereby making it easier to get an excellent night's rest. It is important to train during your daytime hours frequently however, avoid exercising at night prior to bed, as it will cause you to have adrenaline flowing through your body which is not the ideal ambience or the right conditions for sleep. The most effective rule of thumb is to not exercise for more than four hours prior to going to getting to bed.

Think Comfort
Are you comfortable in your bed? If not, make it so! Your mattress should be comfy, and your pillows should too. Make sure your sheets are just just enough to cover you, but not too much and not too rough too. It is also important to be aware of the clothes you put on before your bed. Are you comfortable? Avoid wearing anything that is too tight, and stay clear of anything that can be irritating to your skin. Consider loose and baggy comfy, breathable and don't constantly think about style!

Do not eat before bed
Do not consume food for at least six hours prior to when you sleep. This will make sure that your body has digested your main meal, and won't to give you gas, indigestion or heartburn.

They won't aid in sleeping! Additionally, avoid any product with caffeine in it, since this is a stimulant and can keep you awake, and not aid in a sleepy night. Avoid consuming the coffee before going to bed If you truly require something, choose warm milk.

You can kick your pet out of Bed!
If your pet is sleeping in the same room with you, it could be beneficial to switch it up and make them sleep in a separate room. If they're shifting around and you're sleepy then you're likely to awake and struggle to get back to the sleep. Naturally, if you have infants who sleep in the same room with you, it's not feasible to move them around in the moment But what about pets? They're gone!

Beware of smoking
Smoking cigarettes is harmful in many ways But did you know that smoking cigarettes can cause insomnia as well? The reason is that smoking, i.e. nicotine is a stimulant which means that the longer you take a puff during each day, greater levels of nicotine you'll find within your body. It's common knowledge that smokers are more

difficult to fall asleep. They typically wake up more frequently in the night and their sleeping pattern gets affected as a consequence.

Write it all down
A major and irritating aspects of being on the threshold of sleep and then waking up it's because you've been being too focused, or being too busy with your mind. Stress is the main that causes sleep disturbances and it's likely the scenario that you're sitting in your bed, contemplating everything you've been thinking about throughout the day. You think of things you'd like to take action on the next day to make things better. You begin to worry about the possibility of forgetting the thing that you've decided is the solution to all your problems And from there, you can't sleep without the anxiety. The solution? Keep a pen and a piece of paper on the side of your bed. When you are able to recall something and you are certain you won't want to forget about it note it down on paper and take it off your mind. Repeat this process whenever something comes into your head. Writing down things helps clear our minds of them, and lets us be

able to shut off more quickly.

If you're someone who is prone to planning, i.e. you prefer to make an outline of what you'll accomplish the following day make time at night to write everything down. This will take away one item to think about.

Reboot and try again
If you're having trouble getting to fall asleep and have been lying there for a while without any sleep getting in the way Don't get caught up in it. It will only make the situation more difficult. Instead take a break and do something that's will relax you and help you sleep without overloading yourself. Go through another chapter in your book, play some relaxing music or soak in a warm bath. When you feel your eyes get heavier, do it another time.

Keep a Sleep Diary
It's not just to present to a doctor in case you need to tell them how difficult it is to fall asleep, but it's an extremely useful tool for finding patterns. Record what you did during the day, including what you ate and what you

consumed as well as the night you fell asleep when you awoke up and any worries or thoughts you were experiencing throughout the night. Keep this journal for a few weeks, and then go through it. Do you notice any patterns? Are there any patterns that has a pattern?

In this case, for instance, you could start to notice that once you consume certain foods for dinner, even though you wait six hours before bedtime in accordance with the recommended time but you are still finding it difficult to go to sleep. It could be due to an intolerance to food or sensitivitythat could be affecting your sleep. It could be that you are having trouble digesting the particular ingredient in your food and you are waking up with bloating or heartburn. You may not be aware of it until you record your journal and notice the patterns. Of of course, when you go to your doctor for your insomnia, the sleep journal will also prove very beneficial for aiding them in determining how serious your insomnia is and in helping them identify any patterns that are more difficult to detect to the non-trained eye.

Recognize Your Stress Levels

Stress is a problem and that if you let it to get to the point of extreme it will lead you into health issues that are serious. It's important to note that this can affect your sleep as well. Are you stressed? A lot of people are stressed, and they don't realize that they are. If you are operating with a high degree of stress for a prolonged amount of time it can become normal to you even though you're far from being normal!

Allow yourself to be able to see the extent to which you could in your heart declare that you're stressed out. Then, you can try to discover how stressed. This will give you methods to decrease the stress level and hopefully, it will help you get rid of your sleep problems too.

Consider this in this way: If your mind isn't at ease enough that you can let go all that happened during this day How are you going to go to sleep? It's nearly impossible. It's like laying down following a fight or when you're concerned about something and it's impossible to think of anything else but the issue, and you're just so overwhelmed by it that your mind can't slow down. When you're feeling stressed, exactly like when you're angry and trying to concentrate even the tiniest tasks can be difficult.

The management of stress will definitely help to reduce your sleepiness in this situation. The basic principles of stress management are:

• Discuss the issue that you are experiencing regardless of how minor you may think it is If you require assistance do not feel as if you're refusing to seek help. It's an affirmation of strength to tell someone that you need help, as you'll be able to recognize the incident and not attempt to hide it and likely putting yourself in an even deeper hole
* Exercise regularly This will improve your spirits and help maintain perspective
Eat healthy Doing excessive amounts of the wrong item isn't going to benefit digestion, or isn't going to lead to the most peaceful sleeping habits as well. Additionally you're not providing your body the energy it requires to combat

stress, if you load your diet with excessive sugar and fat

Relaxation techniques are a good option. It's the same in attempting to fall asleep in a natural way, however If stress is the primary sleep trigger, then you'll see that relaxing is a great way to sleep.

Many people suffering from insomnia discover that by altering their lifestyle and habits of sleeping the issue tends to resolve itself quickly. These self-help strategies aren't too complicated, however they provide you with the necessary tools to implement effective adjustments to your routine. Also, you will notice that a lot of these methods are healthy lifestyle practices as well, meaning that it's not just that you'll benefit from better sleeping and better health, but you'll observe that you are feeling healthier overall.

Herbal Remedies to try

Complementary medicine, i.e. herbal remedies and supplements are long-standing and effective alternative to many who suffer from various ailments. Sleeping disorders are certainly one that could be helped by herbal remedies. However, prior to attempting any kind of supplement or treatment similar to this, examine it with your physician. This warning was mentioned briefly before but it's important enough that we have to make sure we reinforce this. It's as simple as one visit to your physician and discuss your issue as well as what you're planning to try. After that, he or can provide you with an answer that is either yes or no and give you suggestions on the most effective herbal remedies you can test.

To be completely honest in our discussion of the various types of treatments for insomnia Let's look at some of the most sought-after and efficient herbal remedies and supplements to insomnia.

Valerian Root
Numerous studies have been conducted on the effectiveness of valerian root on sleep disorders and have all produced positive outcomes. However, as when it comes to any natural remedy, it's hard to determine if it's will work

for everyone around the globe!

Valerian root may interfere with other medication, and it is important to consult your physician prior to you begin using this particular remedy or supplement. There are a few adverse consequences of valerian root but they are not serious and must be evaluated in terms of the pros and cons in relation to your insomnia.

Chamomile
We've all heard about the natural sedative properties of chamomile, which is why it is often used to treat insomnia . If you're allergic to or sensitive towards chrysanthemums and ragweed, stay away, but aside from that, chamomile is an beneficial herb. It is possible to consume it as a tea or take it as an supplement. Many people prefer a spray mist of the mixture of chamomile or lavender that is then breathed into produce similar effects.

Lavender
Lavender is a remarkably similar plant to chamomile it is a natural relaxant and potential sedative properties. Lavender can be consumed

in tea, as a mist, or be used as a massage oil with essential oils. This is a highly versatile and effective herb that it's not just to treat insomnia and anxiety, but also for stress and general relaxation.

A variety of Herbs to try
There are a variety of other plants that are believed to have sleep-enhancing properties, such as hops, passionflower, and lemon balm. They aren't completely proven as of yet, but there's evidence to suggest there is a substantial number of uses for these herbs. If you decide to test the remedies or not is your own individual decision, but be aware that no remedy is completely proven to be beneficial for the individual. We all have our own unique needs and react to various solutions in various different ways.

Melatonin
In essence, melatonin isn't an herb it's a hormone that is produced naturally within the human body and in the plants. Melatonin plays a crucial role to play in the regulation of sleep patterns and sleep in helping the body to know

when it's time to wake up according to the regular body clock. Additionally, this hormone has been shown to be effective for other ailments that could cause heart issues, as well as aiding with jet time. The great news is that melatonin has been recognized as a treatment for insomnia. It is available as supplements.

Talk to your doctor on the best way to take Melatonin however, generally speaking, you should to make sure you are taking your dose at the exact times each day, so that it can get into your body and then become efficient. The dosage you choose to take must be precise, as certain supplements can increase the Melatonin levels in your body too significantly! A visit to your doctor will assist you in determining the proper dosage for your needs and ensure that this kind of supplement is safe in the same way.

Acupuncture
It's it isn't a supplement, but a different therapy technique which has proven to be very effective. There's no place to include acupuncture in this list, so we'll put it here so

that you have the correct amount of details!

Acupuncture is an ancient form of Chinese treatment and is extremely beneficial in the treatment of insomnia. If you're not a lover of needles, then this isn't the ideal option for you. However, If you're not averse to needles and you can tolerate them then you might find relief by trying this type of treatment.

Acupuncture is the practice of using needles that are placed into specific pressure points on the body. In some instances, certain forms of acupuncture may also involve electrical stimulation in conjunction with. By stimulating these points it is believed that acupuncture allows the flow of energy to be more fluid to unblock any blockages and permit sleep to take place in a more relaxed manner.

Each of these remedies, along with some of them are proven to be effective in varying degrees of effectiveness for treatment of insomnia. It is certainly worth giving these remedies a go, but make sure you talk to your doctor first. It could be possible that with specific changes to your sleep habits you will be able to resolve your insomnia issue easy indeed.

Chapter 18: You're Not Alone

If you're in the suffering from a disease that is of any kind it could appear as though that you're the sole person on earth who is suffering at this exact moment. But that's not the case for any kind of disease, since there are likely millions of people around the world who are in the exact vessel like you. However, if you're in a coma at 3am in the morning it's a lonely time indeed.

There are numerous reasons to this which we've discussed a few of them in our previous chapters. However, we could certainly place many of the blame at the feet of our hectic lives, which is the reasons why a lot of us have trouble getting a restful night's rest every night. We've spoken a lot about anxiety and money worries, but what about financial concerns? How many of us lie in bed at night, doing calculations trying to survive? A lot of people do! How many of us are thinking about the 'what ifs and 'what ifs' that are abounding in the world? This is another thing we seem to be unable to do in these times.

The demands of our lives influence our lifestyle, and it also impacts how we sleep. It's not as simple to simply say "okay, let's take a break as our work schedules aren't allowing us to take a break, and our never-ending to-do list isn't likely to shrink just by relaxing and reducing our time! It's a vicious cycle in several ways, but to feel more confident that you're not the only person suffering from sleeplessness, these are the issues that you could keep in mind and encourage yourself in this regard. However, it won't aid in solving the problem but it could make you feel better moment!

The prevalence of Insomnia in our society of today

Insomnia is a problem that affects millions. To provide you with an idea, take a look at some of the statistics.

Researchers at the University of Warwick discovered that 150 million people around the world suffer from problems with sleep frequently. That's a large number of people who toss and turn at night, that's roughly 30percent of globe's population!

The below statistics may surprise you as well:

* On average we (the people in general) are sleeping around 20 percent less than just a century ago.
* One of every three people will experience an insomnia-related disorder of some sort throughout their lives.
* Anxiety and stress (either either or both) is among the most common causes of sleeplessness for Americans More than half the population struggling to sleep.
* There are many reasons why the women of our society are more likely be suffering from insomnia than men and have a double likely to suffer from it.
* Although it is not a proven connection exists, it is believed that an inborn predisposition to insomnia may be the case, since approximately 35% of people suffering from insomnia do have had a history of insomnia in their families.
* People suffering from depression will likely be suffering from sleeplessness at some point and

approximately 90% of those suffering from depression experiencing insomnia

* It is believed that around 10 % of US citizens take some form of sleeping medication. There's a connection between the effects of insomnia on weight gain and obesity, which increases the risk of a sleep-related problem, known as sleep apnoea.

* A poll conducted by the National Sleep Foundation showed that approximately 60% of the people polled have said they have been being tired while driving and tired, with 37% were unable to sleep while driving at one point or another.

* The most common reason behind low sex drive is fatigue

The facts and figures mentioned are truly shocking when you consider the enormous problem that sleepiness is the main cause of insomnia in our modern society. The fact that so many confess to driving while exhausted is alarming as is the percentage of drivers who admit that they doze off while driving is more alarming. The large number of people who require sleep aids prescribed by doctors in the

US exposes the issue to a large extent and the problems that insomnia brings, e.g. anxiety and depression as well as obesity, weight gain and sleep apnoea are all things to keep in the back of your.

When you look at those figures, do you think that you're not alone in your sleeplessness problem?

No!

The Known Sufferers of The Limelight

Naturally, the suffering of the stars is not far from our thoughts, but realizing there are some favorite and beloved stars have the exact issues as we do, helps us realize that they're the same like us, so whatever we're dealing with isn't something that we should confront alone. Some of the following celebrities have confessed to having insomnia in the past

* George Clooney
* Michael Jackson
* Jessica Simpson

* Marilyn Monroe
* Madonna
* Miley Cyrus
* Heath Ledger

Naturally, celebrities lead lives that are chaotic much often, with lots of travel, stress and possibly having to be away from family often. This all ties into the possible causes of sleepiness in general, and emphasize the frequent occurrences.

Although insomnia isn't something that we usually discuss over dinner, you just need to conduct a straw poll of your coworkers in the workplace, or people you see regularly for dinner on an ongoing basisto discover the other members of your social circle has insomnia too. Most likely, at least half will be open about this issue, and it could be an excellent way to meet people who are who are in your corner. A friend who is an insomnia ally can assist you in talking about your issues and help you to release any issues or concerns that are the cause of your insomnia. While it may not work for everyone, it's definitely worth the effort, isn't it?

117

In the following, final section, we'll bring everything together and we'll be sure provide you with some helpful websites to explore regarding the topic. These websites can provide you with additional self-help strategies, as well as details about the subject, and help you connect with professionals who are able to speak to you in case you're looking for additional assistance and assistance.

Don't Let Snoring Steal Your Sleep
The act of snoring can deprive the bedmate or yourself of sleep. It's actually one of the most significant sleep-stealing habits of all.
There are a few ways and products that aid in reducing the effects of average storage. If your snoring is that it is causing your bedmate to be kicked out of your bedroom or even when the door to your bedroom is shut, consult your physician about sleep apnea.
For us we may need to know that we're not the only ones. A recent study revealed that more than 58 percent of couples say that the habit of snoring can cause problems in their relationship!

If you're a victim of your partner's snoring which makes you sleepy (while the other sleeps peacefully) the best option could be to use earplugs for you. I love the silicone ones which can be made to fit in all ears.

If you're the culprit , or have a partner who is willing to listen to your suggestions There are some products you can explore.

Take note of the sound

I am a huge fan of my Sleep Talk Recorder app in the iTunes and Google Play stores for a dollar. Record your snoring at it's worst and let your companion be aware of how loud the snoring is. Android users can download an app called the Smart Voice Recorder application free of charge.

Be aware of the sound

Snoring doesn't sound similar. It differs based on the vibrating of soft tissue in the back of your nostril (pinched noise from your nose) or at the top and back in your mouth (louder or throaty sound).

The reason for this is that the muscles that open the airways relax and tissues become more sloppy and can block the air passageway.

How to stop snoring? Visit the DENTIST. If you notice that snoring is occurring when your tongue falls in the rear of the airway and prevents airflow to the lunges, then the most effective solution is to use a mandibular repositioning device.

The device moves the jaw and tongue forward in order to expand the airway and increase the flow of air. It should be constructed and fitted by a dentist , or an orthodontist.

Lose weight. Obesity is the main reason for snoring, as having an overly fat neck strains the airway, stifles muscles and pushes the tongue to the back.

Make changes to your routine. Alcohol consumption at night relaxes your muscles and is a depressant, and can cause irritation to the airways, which can make snoring more difficult. Certain medications can make snoring more severe therefore ask your doctor or pharmacist about any interactions.

Turn around. It is more likely when you lie with your back against the wall (as numerous of your bedmates will attest) therefore some people manage through sewing tennis balls to on the inside in their pajamas. Learn to sleep on your back.

AWARENESS CHANGES IN MENOPAUSE. It can transform a peaceful sleeper into the sleep snoring machine. The estrogen level of women during premenopausal years and naturally larger, airways can provide protection.

However, as estrogen levels fall the muscles lose their strength and snoring can be more common.

Solutions available over-the-counter

SPRAYS FOR THROAT. These are helpful to some people and are cheap enough to test. A lot of them contain peppermint and other essential oils that help soothe and smooth the throat's back.

NASAL STRIPS. They are placed on the nose's outside and , like the sprays, can be tried for a small cost. I have friends who claim to have reduced the volume of their spouse's snoring.

A ANTI-SNORING STRAP AND CHIN. The cushion is firm and elevates your chin from your chest, which is supposed to open the airways, reducing the amount of snoring. The chin strap was designed to accomplish the same thing. There isn't anyone I know who has tried either successfully.

ACUPRESSURE Anti-SNORING RING. It's likely to sound the most ridiculous of these options however I've seen people who are in love with it. It's not sure if it stops the snoring, but it does for some people decrease the amount.

Know that Snoring is a health Risk
Snoring can result in sleeping problems for the sleepers as well as their bed-mates. It can go from being an issue to becoming an health risk if the snorer ceases breathing for long periods of time.
Sleep-disrupting breathing pauses during the night are afflicted by sleep apnea. Studies have revealed that it affects as much as 4 percent of men , but only one per cent of women.
What are the signs for sleep apnea?
People who suffer from sleep apnea do not have any memories of sleep interruptions, but they rarely believe they've had an adequate night's rest. People with the condition may experience breathing difficulties and tiredness, sleeplessness headaches, depression and fatigue.
Many people snore, however if your snoring

could be detected through a closed door You should consult your physician.

What is the reason it's an enigma for health? It triggers an increase in blood pressure which could increase the speed of tightening and hardening arteries, which increases the risk of suffering a stroke. Don't believe that this is only something to be a problem; it's actually an illness needing treatment.

Do you have a test to detect sleep apnea? There are two common medical tests that could be used to determine the diagnosis such as a cardiovascular MRI (magnetic image resonance) scan or Angiogram, where the radioactive dye gets injected in the arteries of your body to look for signs of thickening of arteritis on an X-ray. Both tests assess how sleep apnea affects you. The most commonly used diagnostic methods However, the most commonly used diagnostic techniques include sleep studies, whether at an inpatient facilities or at the home.

If you're being referred to a sleep facility and you're connected to equipment that is monitoring the heart, lung and brain activity as well as breathing patterns, leg and arm movements , and blood oxygen levels during your are asleep. This is known as the nocturnal polysomnography.

A different option is to use a sleep test kit at home. It is a simple matter of placing an air-flow sensor tube in your nose, place it on an elastic belt and clip an attachment to your finger prior to bed. The sensors test you heart rate, your blood oxygen levels as well as your air flow patterns. If you suffer from sleep breathing problems, the test will indicate a drop in the level of oxygen in the event of sleep apneas (stoppage breath). The test is packaged up with equipment and return it to the lab, which will then send findings to you physician. The positive side is the fact that insurers typically cover these tests, however, they will often require the test at home first before they approve a sleep center. This is because the at-home test is priced at least hundreds of dollars, while testing at a sleep center costs hundreds of dollars.

In both cases the doctor must start the testing and also provide a prescription form for at-home tests.

Treatment options

If you've been diagnosed as having sleep apnea

there are many treatments available.
Treatments that are approved by insurance or medical professionals

Continuous Positive Airway pressure is the one you've heard of. It's basically a mask that which you wear before you go to bed. There are a variety of types and sizes of masks, so you'll have to consult with your physician and CPAP provider to determine the best one for you.

If you've ever experienced scuba gear, then you're aware of what you can expect. It is attached through tubes to an air pump that delivers pressurized air to your nose. The flow of air keeps the airway in the upper part of your nose open and helps prevent the development of apneas.

Around 60 to 70% of patients suffering from sleep apnea are treated using CPAP. It's not a fun experience, but it could be life-changing. CPAP masks can also be loud, which might not be a good thing for the bed partner. Try different models to determine the variation in the sound quality. Insurance plans usually include these features and the costs can vary from hundreds of dollars up to $5,000.

NASAL PATCHES, also known as PROVENT

THERAPY are becoming more popular due to the fact that many patients, in some studies that as high as 50 do not like wearing the bulky masks during the night , and then stop wearing their masks.

In 2008 it was in the year 2008 that the U.S. Food and Drug Administration approved the use of disposable nasal patches. They are reminiscent of Dr. Scholl's corn pads. However, instead of feet, you apply one patch to each nostril with an adhesive made of hypoallergenic.

They are identical to CPAP as they cause pressure in the airways to prevent the airways from collapsing while asleep.

The problem of these patch is they do not fit everyone like CPAP that, when used correctly it is 99.99 percent efficient. Some insurance companies do not cover these , and the cost for a 30 day supply is approximately $200.

DENTAL APPLIANCES could be appropriate for moderate to mild Apnea sufferers.

The dentist will take impressions, either physical or digital, of your teeth. They then send these models over to the dental laboratory in which your customized appliance is designed. They are referred to as Mandibular Advancement Devices (MAD) These look similar to the mouthguards that athletes wear. A little less popular than MAD is the tongue Retention Device, that helps to hold the tongue in place , keeping an airway wide.

The retainer-like devices allow for the opening of your airway through pushing the jaw forward. Many people are less invasive than CPAP masks.

Remember that only a doctor is able to determine if you suffer from sleep apnea. You must be referred to a dentist by your physician when the traditional CPAP or nasal patches don't fit your. Many insurance plans will accept these devices.

SURGICAL INTERVENTION is a drastic treatment option that is typically only advised for patients suffering from more serious problems such as a tonsil polyps, or nasal polyps.

The procedure could involve surgery to the jaw's lower part, which involves removing soft tissue from behind of the throat reducing tissues in the nasal passage by using radiofrequency, or altering the way the tongue is connected.

Alternative treatments

You can play a wind instrument such as clarinet, flute bagpipes, or the didgeridoo. Researchers believe that the breathing technique that is required for playing wind instruments helps strengthen the muscles required to keep your airways clear while you rest.

In a study that was published in British Medical Journal, 25 patients suffering from sleep apnea engaged in the game of the didgeridoo around 30 minutes each day, seven days each week, for four months , significantly decreased the amount of sleep apneas that they experienced in their sleep. The amount of sleepiness during the day also decreased. You can buy a dogeridoo from Amazon.com with under $30.

SWITCH MEDICATIONS. Antihistamines, muscle relaxants , and painkillers can reduce breathing and relax airways, which can makes apnea more likely. If you are taking any medication during the night, ask your physician if they cause your breathing problems. It could be possible to take your medication at a later time or switch to a different one.

Do You Experience Sleepless Sundays?

A lot of people struggle to fall to sleep on Sundays. In fact, an Australian study found that up to 60 % of those affected.

It is true that the biological cycle of sleeping and waking up shifts during the weekend. This is compounded by using the Sunday night as a time to contemplate or fear the coming week. It's difficult to fall asleep with all the brain activity happening.

Our bodies are awestruck by routines, and when we sabotage this routine, it affects our difficulties with sleep.

Tips to help make Monday mornings simpler

Take a light, nutrient-rich carbohydrate dinner in the early hours of the morning. Stay clear of alcohol and sweets.

Get a hot shower or a relax in a bath to cleanse your body.

Wear your pajamas approximately an hour before the time you go to bed to make your brain know that it's the right the right time to turn off.

Sleep in the evening at the same time as your normal workday.

Take away electronic devices emitting blue light out of your bedroom.

Maintain the bedroom at a moderate temperature. The goal is 68 degrees Fahrenheit.

Relax and let your mind wander but don't think about trying to fall asleep. Consider a song you love while letting the words float through your mind.

Don't look bleary-eyed on Monday mornings. The time we spend sleeping and staying up on weekends affects how well we sleep. Plan a bit prior to Sunday night, and you'll be able to avoid the unhappy Monday morning crowd. One company that makes skincare products conducted an analysis of women. They discovered that 20 percent of women who had a bad night's rest on Monday hit an unsustainable level by Wednesday. They appeared older and had lower levels of energy and were stressed more in comparison to those who were sleeping normally.

Don't Be Fooled by Old Wives Tales
Avoid exercising prior to bedtime. It can keep you awake.

It's true that even intense exercise isn't causing problems for the majority of people, in accordance with The Sleep Council.

The method is to slow down by stretching and relaxing when you're done working out.

Relax and close your eyes for several minutes as you take deep breaths and relax your body and mind. relax. If you exercise, do this immediately after when you're planning to exercise next or following an icy bath or shower.

If you are having trouble getting to sleep, you should go to sleep earlier.

This is not a good idea. Sleeping on your back and not getting sleep can cause insomnia. It is better to get active throughout the day to ensure you're not exhausted at the time you're ready to fall asleep.

It is possible that you only require just a few hours of sleep. Everyone is different.

There's a bit of truth in this, but the majority of people are in need of at least seven or eight hours of sleep.

Based on a study conducted by the University of (San Francisco) California, some people have a mutation in their genes which causes them to require only 5 to 6 hours in the night to sleep.

The study only covers 5 percent of the population, but don't be planning any marathons of late-night TV.

Sleeping in for an hour every night isn't going to hurt you.

TV physician and the author of The Fast Diet, Dr. Michael Mosley discovered during an experiment that individuals who had just an hour more sleep than usual schedules had trouble with tests of metal agility the following day.

The worst part is that after a week, their blood tests showed that the biological processes that are associated with inflammation, immune responses and stress were more active. If people slept an extra hour this process reversed.

Don't allow your bedtime to be delayed as you watch this show or read that book. You'll need to get more sleep.

Men require more sleep than women.

In reality, women suffer from more insomnia, and require to get at minimum of each night to rest according to the British Sleep Research Center. Researchers speculated that men are more direct and women are multi-taskers;

hence their brains require more sleep at night. If you're unable to get enough sleep in the middle of your week, you can make amends during the weekend.

However, the reverse is also true. Studies on sleep show that disrupting your body's circadian rhythm causes you to be less able to sleep on a weeknight.

It's fine to go to more early than usual in the event of a rough night prior to. But don't create a routine. You must make it a habit for your body to go to sleep and get up at the right time. Don't take a nap throughout the daytime. It can make you feel more exhausted.

It's all about the length of time you take a nap it's not about how long you rest, but whether you actually nap. A nap lasting between five and 20 minutes allows your brain to relax and help you keep going throughout the day.

There are two caveats:

1.) Do not nap for more than 20 minutes. After that your brain could go into a deeper sleep, which could cause you to feel groggy when get up.

2.) Do not nap at 3 p.m. since this is the time that a normal person's melatonin levels begin to increase, signaling the brain that it needs to be slowing down. Doing so can disrupt your sleep.

Are Sleep or something else making You Tired? Sleeping less is the obvious solution But there are other things that can contribute to the problem.

Depression and anxiety

It's the primary cause of insomnia that, it makes you feeling tired and unfocused, which increases depression.

Take advantage of the simple solutions of eating healthy and exercising each day, even if it's only an hour of walking. If you don't own an animal, think about buying one. Being required to take Fido to the park every day will take you away from the house and help you connect with other dog owners , and provide you something to consider.

If this approach isn't working consult your physician. There is a chance that you will require a specific type of treatment or be reacting to medication you're already taking. For instance, painkillers containing beta blockers, codeine and certain antihistamines may result in fatigue.

Thyroid gland that is underactive

One fifty women are affected by this condition at some point. Nearly every postmenopausal woman that I've met (including me as well as Hillary Clinton) is on thyroid medications, and you're not the only one.

The thyroid hormone is a key factor in the metabolism of our body and low levels cause dry skin and a feeling of coldness, constipation and weight increase. Luckily, it's easy to diagnose with a blood test and managed with a daily pill.

Type 2 diabetes

It is becoming more common for people who are over 40 years old. The reason is due to a deficiency of insulin that moves sugar from blood to the tissues to create energy. Alongside fatigue you may be more susceptible to eye infections and blurred vision and frequent urine leaks.

Diagnostic tests for diabetes require fasting blood tests and treatment could include changes to diet and medications.

Iron deficiency

Iron assists red blood cells transport oxygen throughout the body. Insufficient levels cause anemia that causes fatigue and a lack of breath. It's detected through an examination of the blood and treatment could be iron supplements or changes to your diet like taking in more red meat.

Syndrome of restless legs

If you experience a aching feeling, prickly or crawly in your legs or an overwhelming urge to walk even when sitting still, you could be suffering from the syndrome of restless legs. Your doctor must find the cause of the problem for the issue, such as iron deficiency thyroid problems, diabetes, or adverse effects of a medication you're taking. Treatment usually involves medication.

Your environment

We've discussed the importance of a quiet, cool bedroom. It's also a matter of noise. If you're living within Manhattan or similar cities, there's little that you could do to reduce the outside sounds. I am sorry for apartment dwellers who are in the hands the neighbors.

There are other things which can be helpful. If you own your house put in double or triple-paned (if you are in close proximity to or near an air terminal) window to reduce out outside noise.

If you're a tenant or don't have the money to pay money on new doors or windows Try an earphone or app like the White Noise Free to block outside sounds or earplugs made of silicone available at any drugstore.

Poor air quality can contribute to asthma or allergies which disrupt your sleep. There are air purifiers available for purchase. A few people find relief by keeping a fan running in their bedroom throughout the throughout the night. Make sure not to point the fan at your face or make use of a ceiling fan however, because they can dry your sinuses, which can cause headaches, sinus infections. They can also cause sleep disturbance.

How to Regain Sleep
Don't be worried
Don't get caught up in your problems or allow yourself to become angry at the person or thing. Do not think about what you would like to do to return to your sleep.

Refresh your mind. You can try singing along to a tune you like or mentally chanting the mantra. Simple as saying "ohm" over and over can help you sleep.

Another great technique is keeping a notebook on your bedside table. If something comes to your head you'd like to not forget, record it to make sure your body will be able to relax. If you are constantly thinking of a problem record it with notes that you'll work on it later.

The act of shifting your worries into a journal can cause your body to fall asleep and sleep. Don't watch your clock.

The most stressful thing for insomniacs is nothing more than staring at their clock and wondering the time they'll have to get their sleep. It's not going to ease you to sleep. Breathe deeply.

If you're unable to rest, try to relax. Relax on your back Close your eyes and breathe slowly and deeply , the Pilates method to breathe through your nose, and then breathe out with your mouth.

Tensing your muscles, e.g. your legs, your feet as well as your stomach and arms for a couple of seconds , then let it go. It's not possible to rest until you have released the tension in your body.

Make yourself up and read or catch up on your the television

If tea or hot chocolate helps you sleep, then make yourself the perfect cup. Some people don't like the amount of caffeine found in coco or tea, so you might choose to drink decaffeinated products.

You can read a boring book (not an action novel) or catch the same boring TV show (Home Shopping but which is not The Walking Dead). Relax with peaceful music. Check out the list of apps within

Chapter 19: Media That Help You Sleep chapter.

You're looking to participate in a peaceful, tranquil exercise. This means you should not use a computer or mobile phone, and nothing that could awaken you. Retire to bed after you've yawned.

Don't engage in any activity that you love. You do not want to be rewarded for sleeping less!

Control your environment

You will require a dark and cool,

Be sure that your bedroom isn't warmer than 68 degrees Fahrenheit. Don't wear bulky blankets or pajamas which make you feel too hot. When you're sweaty, it's impossible to be able to fall asleep.

Do not leave blue light bulbs (computer screens as well as other electronic devices) there where you will clearly see them.

This may sound crazy, but I know a neighbor who claims that cooling her pillows helped her fall asleep. The pillowcase is kept in her refrigerator throughout the day, and then puts it on top of her bed before going to bed. This may sound odd but it's free to test.

Learn more about tips in the chapter titled

Control Your Environment chapter.

If you awake at the same time each day Change your routine

If you usually awake at around two a.m. to take a bathroom break and then set your alarm to 1 a.m. You should get up and go about your business.

Retire to sleep and try to keep you eyes open. In no time you'll be asleep. It sounds crazy, but I'm sure it is however, take a chance.

Make use of drugs only as an alternative

In 2011 In 2011, in 2011, the Food and Drug Administration (FDA) approved Intermezzo which is a less-does version of Ambien, which is designed specifically for mid night sleepiness. If your doctor prescribes the medication, he'll certainly inform you of the use. It's not difficult to take a half-asleep pill in the early hours of 2 a.m. Then, you'll forget the medication the medication you took and then try another one at 4. a.m. It's the issue of a hangover if you take a pill in the early hours of 4 a.m. and you have to be up by 6 a.m.

Newer medications like Silenor and Belsomra are believed to cause sleep for shorter durations, and could be more effective than conventional sleep aids. Consult your physician.

Use Drugs
Certain medications can assist you sleep, but not many doctors believe they're as a long-term solution.

Antihistamines
The prescription drugs available such as Benadryl has been utilized in order to promote sleep over a long time. The same components in these allergy medications are found in sleep aids that are available over the counter, like Nytol.

These substances aren't linked to physical dependence, but they can cause psychological dependence.

The issue is that the more you are using them, the more effectiveness diminishes. You might find yourself having to take several pills, and feeling sleepy the next morning because the effects haven't completely worn off.

Melatonin
Another commonly used prescription drug Melatonin is a hormone that regulates your body's cycle of sleep and wake.

A high dose can trigger irritation, restlessness, and sleepiness, so you need to choose the smallest dosage that makes you tired.

Certain people prefer liquid Melatonin. Take two drops of it under your tongue before going to go to bed.

Z and Benzodiazepine

The prescription drugs are Benzodiazepin brands Valium and Ativan and Z-drug brand names Ambien and Zolpidem. Zolpidem as well as Zolpimist.

The drugs function in similarly by altering the way brain chemicals transmit messages to brain cells that are calm.

A variety of potential negative reactions and interactions with other prescription medications including anti-epileptics are present with these medications.

They are particularly problematic for people who are elderly. One study conducted by the U.S. Centers for Disease Control found that excessive use of Ambien caused one out of five emergency Room visits for people who are who are older than 65.

These sedative-hypnotics can cause effects that could make you feel groggy during the day. This can make it easier for senior citizens to slip and fall.

Newer medications like Silenor and Belsomra claim to help you sleep in shorter durations and could be more effective than conventional sleep pills. Intermezzo is a less-does version of Ambien, was developed specifically for mid-night late-night insomnia.

These are the best solution of last resort. However, I know that many older people swear to small doses of Ambien. Consult your physician and learn about the risks to you.

Marijuana

There aren't a lot of long-term studies on the effects of marijuana because, in the past few years, marijuana was banned nationwide and across all states.

At present, 21 states permit marijuana in some form to be used, ranging from limited varieties that are only for medical purposes to recreational use that is open to all adults.

There are anecdotal accounts of people who use it to aid in sleeping.

Another study from 2014 of at the University of Pennsylvania that found the use of marijuana is associated with difficulties sleeping. The participants described difficulty falling asleep and stay asleep but then feeling tired throughout the day.

When marijuana legalized in the state you reside in, consult your physician about using it to help with insomnia. Be aware that the federal government considers marijuana to be a Schedule I substance that has no medical benefits and a high chance of use.

Alcohol

Have any of the 'drugs' been extensively used by so many people for various reasons? The issue in alcohol consumption is that alcohol could assist you in getting to sleep, but drinking too much could cause you to wake up or keep you awake.

In the simplest sense, it may force you to wake up during the evening to go to the bathroom. A lot of people are having trouble getting to the bed.

If someone is doing this every night, evening it can have effects that are in the long run, not just for drinking, but also on sleep disruptions too.

I don't have to bring up the issues of drinking too much alcohol. We've all experienced it throughout our lives for a long time.

Take a glasses of red wine a hot toddy before you go to bed which you can benefit, but don't do not stop at just one.

You can try CBT-I (Cognitive Behavioral Therapy for Insomnia)

In May, The American College of Physicians stated that CBT-I would be able to replace prescription drugs or other aids to sleep as an first treatment for insomnia.

Most people wouldn't argue that non-prescription medications are the most effective solution However, this option can be more appealing in theory than actually implemented. CBT-I was the subject of a media blitz after Sex in the City television actress Kim Cattrall credited it for helping her sleep that was so bad that it forced her to withdraw from the musical in which she was playing.

Technique driven solution

CBT-I actually employs many of the same methods we've explained in this book.

That means creating a tech-free bedroom, and getting out of the bed for a moment in case you're not able to go to sleep after 20 minutes in your bed.

Patients are advised to stay away from coffee after 4:00 p.m. and to eat at least two hours prior to bedtime.

Establish a bedtime as well as a rise time and adhere to the same schedule on holidays, weekends and holiday days.

This is what Mayo Clinic says about it Cognitive behavioral therapy for insomnia is beneficial to everyone suffering from sleep disorders.

For instance, the treatment could help seniors who are taking sleeping pills for a long time, those with physical ailments like chronic pain, and those suffering from primary insomnia.

The effects are expected to last. It is not clear to suggest that CBT-I causes negative side effects.

Insurance can provide coverage for treatment What makes this method different from the advice you'll find the article is that it's customized to the specific patient and requires visits to an experienced sleep therapist for six to eight times over between four and five months.

Many health insurance plans cover these costs and the www.SleepFoundation.org provides a list of trained sleep therapists. If you reside within a city, chances are you have people within 50 miles. If you are in rural or less located areas, you may not have a neighbor. This could be a great method especially if you're dealing with a psychological issue like depression or clinical that's leading to insomnia, or an some physical problem that's underlying, like acid reflux that needs medical treatment. If you think the organization of all these commonly used behaviour techniques into a treatment plan will allow practitioners to charge insurance companies, then you're the same skeptic just like I.

CBT-I has been deemed the best treatment, but certain patients may not like the length of time it takes. Patients who are suffering from insomnia, especially after a significant life event, might not be pleased when they are told to with a therapist for five months rather than the prescription for sleeping pills. Both the doctor and patient need to resolve this issue.

Take a look at Celebrity Tips and Trendy Tips

The Mentalist

Gorgeous television actor Patrick Jane taught the 'count two' method.

Make a mental note of one each time you breathe in, and two when you exhale. Continue to count. You become so immersed in the process that you quit trying to sleep which is the time it occurs.

Dr. Andrew Weil, Prevention magazine columnist 4-7-8 technique

Inhale fully through your mouth.

Shut your mouth, then breathe via your nostrils an imaginary count of four

* Keep your eyes open for seven times

* Breathe deeply into your mouth. Repeat for eight counts.

* Repeat the above sequence three times more.

Craig Ballantyne's 10-3-2-1 formula

* 10 hours prior to bed Do not take any more caffeine

* 3 hours prior to bed: No alcohol or food for 3 hours prior to bedtime.

* 2 hours prior to bed Do not work any more

* 1 hour prior to bed: No screen time

* Zero: The number of times you press the

snooze button during the morning

A trendy exercise for concentration. Lay on your back and breathe deep. Keep your breath in as you contract the muscles on your toes for several minutes. Breathe.

Begin to mentally move your calves. Breathe deeply and then hold your breath. Then, tense your calves for just a few minutes. Breathe.

Begin to move your mind toward your legs. Repeat this procedure until you are at your head. (Actually you'll be sleeping long before you reach your head.)

Advice columnist Ann Landers

Relax in a comfortable position and shut your eyes. Make sure your tongue is away from the ceiling of your mouth as well as your teeth. Relax your tongue until it hangs across the middle of your mouth.

Relax your eyes, then close them. It may take more focus than you'd expect however, do not let your eyes wander.

A few minutes and you'll be sleeping.

Paradoxical intention

Instead of getting frustrated by trying to sleep

attempt to remain awake for as long as is possible. It is not a good idea to ignore your routine or bedtimes you prefer and do not go to bed until you are tired. Sleep in your sleep with your eyes shut and contemplate being awake. Research shows that those who utilize this method are more relaxed than those who do not because it eliminates'sleep anxiety' and makes it easier to sleep better. There's no risk of negative side effects, so it's worth trying.

Sex

The positive side is that sex aids in sleep, decreases blood pressure, and relieves stress. The cuddle hormone is released during the course of sexual activity known as oxytocin. It also reduces the production of the stress hormone cortisol. This puts your body into an euphoric state which allows you to easily sleep. The problem is that sexual relationship must be effective. Ineffective behavior and sexual dysfunction can leave a partner angry and agitated. Be cautious.

Get a complete roundup of the best tips and Tricks

Take a break and enjoy the sun.

A short time in the morning stimulates the brain's release of chemical signals that help to regulate sleep.

Wear wristbands

There are acupressure wristbands available over-the-counter which you can test. It is believed that the same acupressure point in your wrist can prevent nausea and motion sickness is also a great way to relax in the evening.

These bands can be found in any drugstore at less than $10, so it's definitely worth trying.

Utilize the Sachet

A lot of people are in love with essential oils to treat all sorts of treatment. To help you sleep, put lavender sachets on you bedside table. Some sleepers choose to use jasmine over lavender. Jasmine is a great plant for your home. You can keep a small plant on your bedside table.

The fragrant scent of jasmine or lavender activates the regions of your brain which trigger relaxation and reduces blood pressure.

It's possible to put two drops of jasmine or lavender oil to your pillow. It's not harmful.

Download hypnotic CDs to listen to or downloads

The science of Hypnosis has many advocates. There are a few examples of it in chapter Media That Help You Sleep chapter. One study found the reduction of 60% in the frequency of awakenings in the group listening to a sound that soothed the participants to sleep.

See an professional hypnotherapist

Hypnosis is the master's method of letting go and relaxation. A lot of people have tried it to modify their behaviors; e.g., overeating smoking, drinking and getting through different events, e.g. speaking to large groups, giving birth.

In the ideal situation, the therapist will teach you methods to help you relax to sleep soundly.

Make use of a mask to sleep.

I always wear a mask because I've found that the light in my bedroom can make me sleepy. By blocking out light it triggers an increase in the sleep-regulating hormone melatonin. I purchased mine from Walgreens.

It also has a brand new mask known as the GLOtoSleep that resembles foam googles that have blue glow light inside. The mask is held up to an intense lighting for thirty seconds then you put it on.

They are not designed solely to block light, but also direct your eyes up, which can create relaxation brain waves and to focus on the blue light. This helps you rest and sleep.

The reviews for this product are not all positive, however GLOtoSleep is priced at $30 on amazon.com.

Tea drinking

Certain users are devoted to Sleepytime tea made by Celestial Seasonings. Some people prefer the passionflower tea. It is believed that the those teas that contain calming substances can help calm our anxious nerves and allow us to go to sleep.

I have tried a variety of teas, but with none of them producing any results. your mileage could vary.

Make use of Epsom salts to bathe in.

They improve sleep because they increase magnesium levels and aid in the production of serotonin the chemical in your body that aids in relaxation.

You can try one or more of the many natural sleep aids (check with your physician prior to using , and don't mix themup, try each separately to find which one is working for you)

*1 to 3 milligrams Melatonin
* 500-1,000 milligrams of GABA
* 50-200 milligrams of 5 5-hydroxytryptophan
* 150-300 milligrams of magnesium
* 200-400 milligrams of theanine
*365 mg of Magnolia

Find the Top Mattress

Have you ever laid on a bed and discovered that it was worn that you nearly fell across the bed? It's amazing that a lot of people have low mattresses and sleepless complaints to show it. Be aware that firmness isn't the sole indicator of a quality mattress. Be sure to consider the proper size. A large mattress could be sufficient for one person, but two adults and 2 dogs require an king-sized mattress. Don't get one too small; you won't sleep well.

You must be aware of the warranty provided by the manufacturer. The most important thing to consider is the amount that the mattress is likely to sag following usage. Some warranties aren't valid when the mattress is over 1.5

inches. It doesn't seem like much however your back will inform you otherwise.

There is no mattress that will be able to be suitable for everyone. Take a trip to your local mattress stores to test out various kinds and styles. I suggest local stores as the main mattress manufacturers make lines specifically for major department stores like Sears as well as Macys.

When you believe you've got an answer, head back home. Go back to the store on the next day or two and test it again. If it's still not the one then buy it.

Mattresses with different types

SPRING The general rule is the higher the number of springs more springs, the higher the level of support.

The mattress made of box springs is the most well-known mattress one in the U.S. It is made up of coil springs connected to each other that are linked.

In the past, you were told that you should flip the mattress on a regular basis to extend its lifespan. Nowadays, mattresses aren't made to flip , and they only have one side for sleeping on.

This isn't as terrible as it might sound. The mattresses are improved nowadays, and the truth is that when the mattress was wobbly and it wasn't very helpful to flip it around.

POCKET SPRING - Costlier than standard box springs, these springs are small and individual which work in a separate manner. This kind of mattress is ideal when one of the partners is significantly more heavy than the others.

VISCOS ELASTIC OR MEMORY FOAM Thank NASA (National Aeronautical and Space Administration) for its memory foam mattresses that can provide seats with cushioning for astronauts. Memory foam is a good way to distribute your body's weight to provide you with a customized level of comfort and assistance. They can be expensive.

LATEX is hypoallergenic and anti-microbial that makes them perfect for those suffering from allergies. They are also more comfortable than memory foam, so you won't get too hot in the mattress. They can be quite heavy and can vary in terms of quality.

Hybrids - There are many kinds of hybrids on the market like latex and memory foam, memory foam box springs and on and on.

The best option is to go to a mattress store and lay upon the bed. It's also an excellent option to purchase them locally, where the store will collect them in the event that you decide you do not like the mattress or if you spot an issue with the manufacturing. The cost of shipping a mattress and springs back online to an retailer can cost several hundred dollars.

Here are some names

I absolutely love my TempurPedic

It was pricey however I was able to get an excellent deal at Costco.com for a model that is no longer available. I am awed by its firmness as well as the ability to turn over in bed and not disturb my dog or husband and vice versa.

If this or other memory foam mattresses make you too hot, the solution for existing beds is the http://www.coolingmattress.com/ mattress pad. Tempur-Pedic also offers mattresses with a cool top that is incredibly comfortable.

If this brand isn't in the budget, Costco and Sam's Club have lower-cost memory foam options and a number of mattress stores in the U.S.

The Sleep Number option is the preference of many couples

You've probably seen advertisements that demonstrate how a couple can change the thickness and firmness on each mattress (which are actually air mattresses, but are more luxurious unlike the ones you can blow up to accommodate visitors staying overnight) to meet their individual needs. They're not cheap however my daughter and son-in-law are in love with theirs.

I warn buyers that there are mechanical components that could need to be replaced and the bladder that is in the middle could sag in long-term usage. Check out the warranty details at sleepnumber.com before buying to you are aware of what is and what is not covered.

If you think money can buy you sleep, think again.

The luxury mattresses are very popular with the well-off baby boomers. If you're looking for a bed that's affordable take a look at the hand-crafted $644,000 (yes 64,400) Swedish Vividus bed. It is said to take at least 160 man-hours in the making and utilizes natural materials like horsehairs.

If you think that's too much If that isn't enough, the Hastens Swedish firm offers alternative

models that start at $10,000. Visit
http://www.hastens.com/en.

In the same way, it is similar to British competitor, the Hypnos company has a range of beds that range from 10,000 to $30,000. The company provides the beds provider to the British royal family. They also offer the non-royals custom-made beds that are made to be ordered. Visit
http://www.hypnosbeds.com/index.aspx.

If you're looking to work with American firms, the most popular mattress manufacturer is Sealy and offers an extensive price and high-quality assortment of mattresses. Sealy's premium Stearns and Foster line has mattresses that range from $1,000 to $4,000.

Find out the Five Tests to the Best Mattress

1. Relax in your usual sleeping position and then flip over. If your mattress is too soft, it'll take a lot of an effort to rotate. If the bed is too firm it'll cause discomfort on your hips and shoulders.

2. In the event that your bed was designed designed for two people, then both of you

should lay on it for at minimum 15 minutes. You should both try turning before turning back.

3. A friend or partner should be watching you lay upon the bed. If it is supportive and your back, your spine needs to be straight when you're sitting on your side and maintain your normal curve while lying back.

4. If you're lying side on your mattress try to see whether you can slip your hand through the back's hollow. If there's not enough space it's because the mattress isn't firm enough. If your hand is sliding into the bed but your hips or shoulders hurt, it's not rigid.

5. Think about the base you'll place the mattress on, and how high it'll be when considering mattresses. A mattress with a height of 7 inches requires the use of a step ladder, if you purchase a mattress that is thick with box springs.

Where do you place the mattress?

The mattress manufacturer must provide suggestions for the best bases. If you choose a solid base, your mattress will be more firm. A base with slots can provide a more comfortable feel.

I generally suggest looking at a steel frame that

has springs, or even slats. If that isn't for you, consider a different branching out.

I have friends who are adamant about plywood bases, however, it's extremely uncomfortable for your back. Solid surfaces are also not able to permit ventilation, which can in reducing the build-up of mold.

The majority of mattresses work with a power base , however consult the personnel at the store or the manufacturer's site to confirm the mattress you have purchased will work with the base you have.

A few people prefer using frames made of steel and avoid the the box spring. Also, inquire with the store or the site of the manufacturer regarding this. This could cause a warranty to be invalidated.

It is a good idea to purchase your mattress from a store where you are able to exchange it in a fair time of time, if the frame/mattress/no box spring isn't working for you.

If you're not satisfied with the selections at mattress stores, you could consider Ikea which offers the type of slatted bases that are more frequent in Europe.

Get the Linen Closet Stocked Up

Pillows shouldn't be left out

We can go through the process of choosing mattresses and then forget about pillows. You should test a few types to determine the firmness of the pillow you prefer and whether you prefer sleeping with a single pillow or more on top of your head.

The aim is to keep an ideal posture to ensure you do not awake with a stiff neck. This is achieved by keeping an even alignment (shades of the class of Pilate) by keeping your head squarely on your shoulders and not bent to much forward or back.

A few people love this neck cushion (with an opening at the center) however, some dislike them.

If you are allergic then you should stay clear of goose down and other types of feathers. You can also choose pillows that have synthetic stuffing.

It is believed that certain kinds of pillows are best for specific types of sleepers. e.g. Side sleepers need a pillow that is less padded than those who sleep on their backs. The issue is that the majority of us lie on our backs and sides, as well as our backs when we sleep, therefore I don't take these advices take too take too seriously.

I would rather sleep with a hard Temper-Pedic mattress, but you'll have to choose your personal preference. Don't forget that you need a good pillow.

A good place to begin exploring pillows to start is Target. They carry a broad selection and affordable costs.

Certain pajamas are better than others

Satin, silk , or polyester are prone to hold on to your body's moisture and heat. They can cause your bed to be too hot to be comfortable.

Natural fibers like cotton are best.

And, even better There are now sheets and pajamas made of microfiber made to wick away moisture, and let you sleep more peacefully.

Don't be afraid to put your pajamas or bedding in the freezer or refrigerator for 30 minutes to get them cool before you fall asleep. This will assist in relaxing your body.

If you place their sheets frozen for a night and the cold kills dust mites. If that's just a bit hot for you, you can try adding gel ice blocks to your bed, be it those you can freeze and put in your lunchboxes or those you use to treat injuries in sports.

The bedding can aid or hinder sleep

Sheets and pillowcases are available in a variety of materials, from costly linen to inexpensive polyester. Be aware of any allergies you may have and how crucial wrinkle protection is to you.

However they may feel in the shop the sheets will appear different after you wash them before putting them on your mattress. Be sure to keep the receipt for sales until you've tested the sheets both in the washing machine as well as on your bed. You might want take back a product that is shrinking or feels rough after usage.

It is also possible to return the sheets in the event that they aren't fitting properly. It's hard for you to locate sheets that will fit to a California King mattress and cheaper sheets might not been designed with deep pockets.

Sheets to be used as guidelines

Guidelines: Look for sheets that have thread counts that are in the 200-800 range. Above that, you can find more rigid sheets that won't circulate air and could cause you to be too hot. Below are sets that are less expensive which may feel rough once they're washed.

The light colored sheets reflect light rather than absorption, and you would like your bed to be the ideal temperature of 68 degrees Fahrenheit or so.

Don't lie in bed naked, but. A loose cotton nightshirt or pajamas made from natural fibers will remove sweat and help reduce your temperature and make you feel at ease.

Beware of heavy comforters or duvets that could cause you to be too hot and disrupt your sleeping.

Find out What Works for me

What I did when I began to struggle with my insomnia:

I began keeping a nightly journal. It wasn't an attempt to write anything down. It was a simple notebook that I kept in mind to record any thoughts that were distracting me; e.g. the blue light of the charging device or any other thought I couldn't shake off from my head.

If I was concerned about something particular

I'd note it down and then put the possibility of finding a solution in it.

If, for instance, I were worried about a car bill I'd write 'car payment in notepad and then contact a counselor at a credit union on the following day.

For more serious issues I'd recommend writing the problem down, e.g. Find new employment however, the best option could be to simply write out a plan for the following day. It's not a good idea to keep your eyes on the details of your plan.

The idea is to clear your mind from the stress of that subject tonight so that you can sleep. The approach is similar to your Scarlett O'Hara approach, I'll be thinking about it tomorrow. What I do at in the evening:

* Make sure you go in bed around the same time every night (really make an effort).

3. Don't eat food for 3 hours prior to the time you go to bed. (A large meal just before the time of bed will keep me awake.)

Make sure you put on sleep clothes like pajamas, 30-40 minutes before the time of bed. This sends a signal for my brain to signal that it's time to begin slowing down.

Keep the bedroom in a cool and dark place (about 68 degrees Fahrenheit is ideal in my opinion).

Remove any blue screens like smartphones, computers and tablets from your mattress. Do not leave any device plugged in the area where you can see the charger light..

If I feel I'm in need to wind down , before I go to bed, I will:

1. Read non-fiction (no can't-put-it down books) for about 10 minutes or until I feel sleepy. Magazines are ideal to do this. I find it helpful to remove issues that I would otherwise think over and replaces them by thoughts on a simple article.

If I'm having a hard time, I will rise and lie down on my chair as I go through my books. The rocking motion aids me in relaxing. It is believed that rocking can boost the production of serotonin and oxytocin hormones that relax tension muscles.

If I'm in the bed but not sleeping:

I practice the technique taught by Ann Landers. When I shut my eyes, attempt to relax my eyes. My tongue is let free in my mouth, and not touch my tooth or my mouth's roof. I let my tongue hang loose and relax. Sometimes I sing an old tune or lullaby. I'm not sure why, but this is what works for me.

Then it's nighttime.

Go camping

If you're enticed by the television or playing with the phone keep you awake until night, it's the ideal time to pitch your tent out and enjoy the outdoors. Stay away from electronic devices and enjoy an intensive detox every now and then often. Set yourself in a quiet zone and observe your surroundings and yourself. Take this time to think or do some yoga, compose, recollect your thoughts, or unwind. Based on a couple of tests, campers who do not use gadgets and focus to slow down their ceremonies like contemplating or listening to music, fell asleep about two hours earlier than they had anticipated. Another important point to remember is the fact that computers contribute to sleep disturbance. It has been discovered that false light sources could negatively affect the circadian rhythms. Try laying down on from the ground, not inside your car or in a lodge. So, you'll feel grounded and feel a part of the natural world. No matter what you do outdoor activities, the main goal is to relax, free your self from demands and interruptions from other people, stay free of fake light and to be in tune with the natural world. Shower in the normal daylight and then relax when the sun sets. With a snap of imagination, you'll be able to reset your sleep rhythms.

Power Down To Sleep Better
The rest isn't just an on and off switch. Your body requires time to relax and get ready for shuteye. People who haven't slept often believe that it's difficult to shut their minds at evening hours. It is possible to try shutting down and rest better. This method helps to calm things down, with the intention that your body understands that it's the perfect time to take a break. To allow your body to relaxation, it's vital to relax and reduce the psyche. For instance in the event you consume a warm drink prior to bed, it will cause a decrease in your internal temperature, setting the body up to start prepping for rest. Cleaning up your body's heat levels will limit metabolic capabilities such as

absorption, breathing and the pulse. Your body will realize that this is a good time to slow down and relax. In the event that you're prone to listening to music prior to going to the bed every night the body will have trained to recognize that turning on music in the evening is a sign of sleep time.

It's all about the potentialities and shaping. Take at least 30 minutes of wind-down time prior to bedtime for breathing or unwinding exercises to relax your brain. The purpose of this shut-down hour is to remind your brain that this is an ideal time to unwind, slow down and unwind.

Relax In A Cool Room

People who experience difficulty falling asleep generally have a higher internal temperature before sleeping, compared with their more beneficial counterparts. Therefore, this group of people who are restless must remain awake for at least occasion between 2 and four hours until their internal temperature levels come down and they can begin to rest.

The research suggests that the best temperature for a room to rest is between 16 and 20 degrees Celsius. If you're trying to relax your brain, it appreciates the cool climate. Additionally, cool rooms can help in the fight against maturing. It aids in the release of the hormones that mature, namely melatonin which is a powerful cell-based reinforcement that manages irritation, strengthens the fragile framework, prevents intellectual degeneration as well as malignant development. There's a saying that people who go to bed early and wake up early are more likely to live. This suggests that a night of rest in a cool space can reduce the risk of neurodegeneration and increases the pressure of oxidative. I could go on forever with regard to the anti-aging benefits of a good night's sleep in a cool environment. However the best way to boost the development of harmful maturing hormones within your body is to get adequate sleep. Additionally, the first step to achieve this is to achieve a sleeping condition by lowering the temperature of your room. A lack of rest has a number of harmful consequences to the physical and mental health of your. It can also put your life at risk. Therefore, make it a point to improve your sleeping patterns and start doing this by creating the perfect dozing conditions.

Break A Sweat

Get active early. It's an established fact that exercising improves sleep and overall well-being. In any event the examination within the diary Sleep indicates that the amount of exercise is completed as well as when exercise is having any effect. Researchers have discovered that women who exercise at a moderate intensity for in any time period of 30 minutes each morning, seven days a week, have less trouble getting enough rest than women who do earlier or later during the daytime. The morning workout appears to affect our body's rhythms, and increase our quality of rest. One of the reasons for this interplay between rest and exercise could be the internal heat level. Your body's temperature increases during exercise and can it can take as long as six hours to return to a normal level. This is due to the fact that cooler internal temperatures lead to your body's more likely rest. Therefore, it is essential to allow your body the chance to cool off prior to bed. The importance of rest is in the aspect of our health and healing. Take note of it and seek the help from a reputable medical professional in case you are unable to achieve a level of rest. These all need control and responsibility. If you can reset your natural clock, and then return to the routine of musical rest You'll eventually enjoy the benefits of resting in a tranquil, peaceful environment.

Lifestyle Modification to Help Insomniac
In the last portion, we talked about the two primary types of solutions that can be used to combat sleep lack. In reality that these external causes can't deal with the root cause of sleep lack. In fact, you may be more relaxed in the course of studying these remedies however, sleep loss can be completely cured when the source of the problem is eliminated. Another thing to consider is that there is a good chance that a sleep disorder will slide backwards.

What's the basis of sleep lack? For some, the main reason for a sleep disorder is a bad way of living and a tendency to rest. A simple way of living adjustments can greatly improve the quality of your sleep. in the quality of your sleep.

While not all sleep deprivation is caused through pressure, it is known that those who suffer from constant pressure are more vulnerable to overcome a sleeping disorder.

Due to pressure-related insomnia disorder. Treatment or getting rid of the pressure can help alleviate a sleep disorder. In the preceding section of this publication, stress can affect the quality of the resting process, which could disrupt the rhythm of their sleep. Therefore, one may think that it's tough to fall off in the evening and stay alert throughout the daytime. It is crucial to manage all aspects of your daily life in the best possible way so that you're at an appropriate level of equalization. You must ensure that you're getting enough sleep day in and day out.

The importance of rest is for your physical health. If you don't get enough rest, even for a short period of time can make you unhappy and angry. The long-term consequences are not a joke such as heart issues depression, anxiety, stroke and coronary problems, to name a few examples.

According to sleep experts some studies have shown that when people get enough sleep, they will not only feel better, but will also improve their chances of living longer, healthier and productive and ultimately, the sky is the limit once they have achieved their lives. To prevent sleep deprivation it is recommended to stay clear of caffeine, nicotine, or alcohol. They can cause the brain to be anxious after a certain amount of time generally. The constant intake of caffeine can cause the brain to become more active than it currently is. Most people need energy to start their day and so they chose an the energizer. Caffeine is among the most popular choices of energy drinkers today, to guarantee focus and alertness during the beginning of the day, and throughout the rest days. However, they aren't aware of the fact caffeine is among the most significant causes of sleep lack. It can disrupt the typical balance of alertness and relaxation. This is why restless people should stay away from these drinks to get a good night's rest. Do not take a quick nap and go for a glass of plain water instead of the espresso. This could be the reason you're having trouble falling asleep and remaining unconscious until evening time.

In addition making a bed schedule for yourself is the most effective from other methods to improve self-esteem to treat a sleep disorder. It's a major step in fighting sleep deprivation the better. It is crucial to get up and go to bed at night and rise at the same time every morning, as the body requires regularity. The body favors a daily routine. It is thriving with a tendency. If you have a regular sleep and the time to wake up your body is likely to be on the right track. If you're able, stay clear of night-time parties, rotating plans and night shifts or other things that could disrupt your sleep schedule. If you experience some nagging memories sleeping, you can sip an ice cold glass of milk. It's a common remedy for sleep problems and it's been proven that it could help you in getting better sleep. It is not just the case that milk can help keep the urge to eat from disrupting your sleep but it also includes an amino corrosive, tryptophan. This amino corrosive is transformed by the brain into the "unwinding" substance called serotonin. Calcium is an extremely master of metabolism, reducing pressure, and decreasing levels of parathyroid hormone that has been proven to be involved in sleep lack. In addition it is possible to alter your routine to include the time for meditation or yoga. There's a lot of evidence that suggests meditation and yoga can enhance the rest patterns, often significant. Being able to unwind some energy for yourself is important. These techniques should be attainable at home, for comfort and safety. It aids in increasing the limitless ability of your body to adapt as well as relaxes your mind and relieves stress on your body. Try to dedicate at least 30 minutes a day to contemplate or do yoga. Yoga and contemplation are best practiced in the morning hours, in a quiet spot, and in the light of the sun. If you want to reflect, lay down and unwind your mind. Try to listen to a relaxing playlist to calm you. Once you get used to thinking about the day, your psyche will be able to unwind faster in the evening, and you'll have a much easier sleep. In terms of yoga, you could choose to attend classes with lots of other people or at home for greater security. You will benefit by allowing you to see multiple perspectives. The practice of yoga postures can increase the circulation of blood to the most optimal location in the cerebrum which can have the effect of normalizing the resting cycle. Remember, rest isn't an option for living or a luxury It's a necessity and necessary. Find the root reasons, alter your eating schedule and drink a glass hot milk create an evening routine, do some yoga and reflect. Follow the suggestions above and over the long term you'll enjoy a good night's sleep.

Switching Off

How to 'Switch Off' at Night
The first thing you need to do once you've finished eating dinner and tidying down for the night is to shut down any of your electronic devices. If you have your phone or computer

switched on while you're in bed will be arousing experience for your thoughts and eventually hinder your sleep. Be aware that the electronic gadgets you use are addictive and you'll never know the time to turn them off.

The light could interfere with your sleep pattern and will cause you to be in a state of consciousness. It's recommended to stop using your gadgets regardless of time prior to bed time.

It's fine to read before you go to bed but not on your electronic devices. Reading a book in a physical format to relax before going to bed will help you prepare to sleep. It is better not to read within your room. It is recommended to browse in an alternative room because your psyche doesn't have to be active in the space you're forced to be in. Another time, you need to train your brain to switch off when you walk into your space. If you're able to relax while reading an ebook, at that moment, you can read while lying in your the bed. It's also a good idea to read in a different space. Another thing you could do is listen to music and take notes of information you'll require the following day. Music can assist in calming your mind and relieve pressure. Try to listen to music that is more smooth and slower in its cadence. If you are listening to something raunchy or energetic will stimulate your brain and cause it to be more likely for you to fall asleep. In other words you'll find yourself in a more relaxed state by listening to classical music rather than awe-inspiring music. Another suggestion is to plan your rest day prior to the start of your day. Making notes for the next day can help you to get rid of your head.

Being awake and alert in bed continuously telling yourself that you must remember things will keep your mind active. Imagine your scratchpad as an "dump it and forget about the item" vault. You can grab a small piece of paper and write some notes down. This will help you in getting quiet and sleep more quickly.

Another thing you could do is take a relaxing beverage like tea before you go to getting ready for bed. If you do, make sure that you do not drink alcohol, caffeine, as well as drinks with a significant concentration of sugar. A cup of good tea can calm your mind down and help your body to relax. This is also an excellent way to take space for you. It is a chance to unwind and relax. You can do this by browsing or listening to music. If you aren't finding pleasure with tea drinking, this you should consider taking a small snack prior to going to bed. Be careful not to eat any food that is extremely packed with calories and is difficult to digest.

In all cases, a light snack is okay because, sometimes the reason you're having difficulty finding time to relax is primarily due to desire. Another method to ensure a restful relaxation is to reduce the temperature in your room. The best way to achieve that is set your room's inside regulator to be cooler. The body's adaptation is such that when it is in the cooler climate it'll get an indication that it's the perfect time to take a break.

Additionally, why not scrub down prior to going to bed. Ideally , a bath will immediately cool down. Otherwise, you could try to find a bed fan or cooler cushion or go for a quick walk prior to going to bed. The above suggestions can be a part of your sleep routine. You are welcome to test them and determine what is most effective for you and your schedule. In just a few minutes regardless of your imagination, you'll never have any issues with falling asleep and being unable to sleep again.

finally beat it.

Conclusion

I hope this book will help you with stopping or preventing a sleep disorder. It is possible to apply any of the tips and tricks described in this book in order to get an unwinding sleep. In the end, a peaceful sleeping is the basis for your physical and psychological well-being. It doesn't matter if it's a fake or a typical cure, lifestyle modifications, or establishing routines, all of will help in preventing sleep disorder. So what should you do right away? It's a perfect time to take action today! Find out which strategies will work for you, and implement them in your day to daily schedule. Keep them in mind and visualize the way your daily routine will appear like when you incorporate these methods to your routine exercise routine.

If you give these a try and you will determine the best route to conquer sleep disorders.